ENDORSEMENTS

"I give Kelley 5 stars because he has literally saved my life. I was overweight and out of shape, so I decided to try his 30-day challenge. I've lost 25lbs, he really cares about people, and he has shown me different recipes and different ways to curb my appetite. I highly recommend him as he is such an inspiration. If you want to live a healthy, happy, and energetic life, just take the challenge. You will be glad you did!"

—Rodney T.

"Kelley, you are the true definition of a friend. You are definitely the guy that I'd want to have my back in the trenches. Your humor is unmatched, and you inspire me with your accomplishments and there are more of those to come."

—Victor W., US Navy Retired

"Kelley is very knowledgeable in nutrition. He was empathetic towards my desired health goals. He served as a guide through the toughest parts of my journey. I am down 17 lbs in two months after transitioning to a vegan lifestyle."

—Samuel H.

"Kelley is very informative and encouraging. He has helped me in the first 30 days alone reach amazing weight loss goals and all through just following the simple plan that he lays out. I feel and look better. I highly recommend having One Determined Vegan to help you regain your health and to keep you on track."

—Mary G.

"I'm very thankful for having the opportunity to work with Kelley. He provided so much information and assistance from day one. He definitely gave me a lot of direction as for what to eat, and how to make the transition seamless. I would recommend him to anyone who is even slightly interested in giving their body the right fuel."

—Kemari M.

"Kelley has been great to work with! I have been a vegetarian for years and wanted to make the jump to veganism. When I followed Kelley's journey, I knew he was the guy to speak with. He has done so much research and has taught me how to balance my diet for great weight loss results. I'm very happy about making the jump, so if you want to change your lifestyle, Kelley is your man!"

—Heather T.

"If you want to get serious about your health, Kelley can help you achieve that. I was already in pretty good shape. I work out daily and I'm a vegetarian who is used to intermittent fasting. I needed some help to get where I wanted to be and was seriously challenged. But it was so worth it! The amount of energy that I now have, which is why I did the challenge in the first place, is amazing! It is well worth it so go for it because your health depends on it."

—Kailene R.

Plants Saved My Life

*How Going Vegan Transformed
My Health*

Kelley Gilberry, CHN

Plants Saved My Life: How Going Vegan Transformed My Health

Jones Media Publishing
10645 N. Tatum Blvd. Ste. 200-166
Phoenix, AZ 85028
www.JonesMediaPublishing.com

Disclaimer:

The author strives to be as accurate and complete as possible in the creation of this book, notwithstanding the fact that the author does not warrant or represent at any time that the contents within are accurate due to the rapidly changing nature of the Internet.

While all attempts have been made to verify information provided in this publication, the Author and the Publisher assume no responsibility and are not liable for errors, omissions, or contrary interpretation of the subject matter herein. The Author and Publisher hereby disclaim any liability, loss or damage incurred as a result of the application and utilization, whether directly or indirectly, of any information, suggestion, advice, or procedure in this book. Any perceived slights of specific persons, peoples, or organizations are unintentional.

In practical advice books, like anything else in life, there are no guarantees of income made. Readers are cautioned to rely on their own judgment about their individual circumstances to act accordingly. Readers are responsible for their own actions, choices, and results. This book is not intended for use as a source of legal, business, accounting or financial advice. All readers are advised to seek the services of competent professionals in legal, business, accounting, and finance field.

Printed in the United States of America

ISBN: 978-1-948382-54-0 paperback

DEDICATION

This book is dedicated to my mother, Reverend Marcia Jones, who raised me to go after my dreams and groomed me to stand up for what I believe in. You left this world way too soon, but your impact will live on forever! And to my Uncle Walter (Lou) Williams; you also left this world way too soon, but your legacy and story is being told by people that you've blessed and by the hearts you've touched.

ACKNOWLEDGEMENTS

I would like to acknowledge and thank everyone who allowed me to practice on them during my certification phase. To all my friends and family who listened to me during my learning phase, because I know at times it was probably a lot to deal with. I want to acknowledge all my learning resources from the tons of books I've read, researched, and studied regarding health and nutrition. To the many hours of podcasts, interviews, and lectures that I've listened to on the subject.

Thank you to all of those in the plant-based community who have come before me to pave the way which now allows me to have a voice within this space. Their lifelong work and dedication to the mission of natural healing has influenced me to up my game by continuing to learn, to be a sponge! Folks like Dr. Milton Mills, Dr. Michael Greger, Dr. Jeffrey Bland, Dr. Joel Fuhrman, Dr. John McDougall, Dr. Michael Klaper, Michael Pollan, Walter Veith, The Satvic Movement, and many more. To my book publisher, Mr. Jeremy Jones and team, thank you for making the book process such an amazing experience. It is my hope that this book will help someone change their own health outcome for the better, so I salute you! And last but certainly not least, I want to say thank you to my lovely wife for all your support during the writing of this book.

TABLE OF CONTENTS

Introduction: My Story. xvii

Chapter 1: The Laws of Nature 1

Chapter 2: Why Are We SO Sick? 13

Chapter 3: Medicine Isn't Healthcare,
 Food is Healthcare. 29

Chapter 4: Weight Loss 101 39

Chapter 5: The Circadian Rhythm
 (Internal Clock) 51

Chapter 6: Healing Naturally Through
 Plant-Based Nutrition 61

Chapter 7: Did Someone Say Protein? 71

Chapter 8: Marketing is One Hell of a Thing. . . . 83

The Final Chapter: Adopting the Right
Mindset 93

About The Author 101

FOREWORD

I have known Kelley Gilberry for over 19 years. Our friendship developed in the Navy. In the military, you meet a lot of people, you serve with a lot of people, but there are only a select few that you consider a true friend in life after serving your country. Kelley has a great sense of humor and loves to have fun as I do, and we have had great lasting memories over the years. If there is one word to describe Kelley, it would be *passionate!* Kelley has been fervent and dedicated to ensuring a healthy lifestyle, not only for himself and his family, but for anyone he associates with. I have seen the transformation in his life firsthand, and it's extremely noteworthy!

Those that know me, know I love my family, love to have fun, and love to travel, but what good is it to have a love for something if you don't love and take care of yourself in the process! What do you have a love for? What is your "why" in life? You deserve all the great things life has to offer. I know this book will encourage you and get you on the healthy path your life deserves.

Kelley will lay out his testimony, his journey to a healthy lifestyle, and provide guidance to help you live the life you desire, because your life will literally depend on it.

**Rodrequiez (Rod) Holman
(Entrepreneur)**

PREFACE

This book includes all the things I've learned and implemented when it came to totally transforming and regaining my health. As an instructor at the US Naval Academy, I learned what it took to deliver messages in such a way that leaves little room for misinterpretation. In the military, there are times when life and death is dependent upon the decisions being made. Though I am no longer in the military, I still use those same techniques to deliver messages of health and natural healing to my clients, friends, and family. I have been an instructor and teacher for over 17 years, so delivering messages that get straight to the point by cutting through the red tape is what I specialize in. I use lots of stories and analogies to drive home my points, so buckle up, strap in, and enjoy the ride.

Introduction:

MY STORY

In 2021, at the age of 42, I had gone from the worst shape of my life to the best shape of my life by using the power of plant-based nutrition. So, the question is, "what prompted me to make such a drastic change from the Standard American Diet (SAD) for which I had known my entire life to a Whole-Foods, Plant-Based Vegan Lifestyle?"

To understand exactly how plants saved my life, you'll first need to understand the circumstances behind the change. In October of 2019, I received a phone call from my older brother telling me that our mother had gone into the hospital for a routine heart procedure, as she has had issues controlling her cholesterol over the years. He told me the procedure didn't go well, as our mother's heart had stopped beating during the procedure, so the doctors had to revive her to bring her back to life.

I live in Texas, and she lives in South Carolina, so I immediately jump on the next plane going east, because I needed to be by my family's side during such a horrific and scary time. When I arrived at the hospital, my mother was connected to three different life support machines. The doctors came in to tell my family that she was very sick, and the chances of her surviving were not good. So, it would probably be best if we said our goodbyes.

Once we received this news, I just couldn't figure out how to process it, so I walked around the hospital in total solitude away from my family. If you were to know anything about me, it is that I need time to process new information in my own head before I'm able to express "how" I'm feeling towards others. During my walk, I received another phone call from my older brother telling me that I needed to get back to mom's hospital room immediately, because she was getting ready to pass away! So, I rush back to the room just in time to see my family is surrounded by our mother's bedside. I see my sisters crying, my brothers crying, and my father's face filled deep with sadness. The life support machines that I mentioned earlier were no longer able to maintain her weakened heart. I dropped to my knees and the tears flowed from my eyes, because I saw the heartbeats from her rate monitor dropping to zero. Within a matter of 48 hours, I had gone from being extremely happy and excited about my family's future, to a man who was now lost, because his mother was gone! After her funeral, I got back on the plane to fly back home asking myself, "what the hell just happened?" The truth of the matter was my mother had just passed away from a *heart attack,* which is the leading cause of death in the United States.

After returning home, I looked into the mirror and realized I was in the worst shape of my life. You see, I served in the US Navy for 12 years where I was always in pretty good shape because I had to stay within military weight standards. In the Navy, I did four world tours at sea, and the last three years were spent as an instructor at the US Naval Academy in Annapolis, Maryland, where I became a Certified Master Training Specialist. It wasn't until I transitioned out of the Navy and into the real world; that was when all my weight issues began. But what's funny is at the time I didn't realize how out of shape I was; I had no idea that I was losing my health. It wasn't until I went in for a routine doctor's visit shortly after the passing of my mother, that I realized my health had spiraled out of control. I received the news at this very same visit that I had both prediabetes and a condition known as "angina," which is basically an early warning sign that a heart attack is lurking right around the corner. That diagnosis hit me like a ton of bricks. Keep in mind my mother had just passed away from a heart attack.

About five or six months later in early 2020, around the time COVID-19 introduced itself to the world, my mother came to me in a dream and told me that I have the God-given ability to help others heal. I had absolutely no idea what that dream meant considering I was in the worst shape of my life, and considering my recent diagnosis of two chronic diseases. I said to myself, "I don't know anything about healing, so how can I help others heal?" But as the days and weeks passed, no matter how hard I tried, I could not seem to shake this powerful dream. Well, about a month after having this dream, my wife and I received the news that her favorite uncle, who practically raised her, was given only two months to live, because the cancer that he had once beaten is no longer in remission and it's back with a vengeance.

Of course, this was devastating news for us, so the family decided to have him live with my wife and I, because the place where he was receiving his treatment was practically in our backyard. You see, we live in Houston, Texas, which is the place where the well-known cancer hospital MD Anderson is located. My wife worked on a nursing schedule, so she was doing a lot of shift work. I was able to work from home because everyone was ordered to stay at home until the world figured out what to do about COVID-19. Therefore, I was able to take him to his daily and weekly doctor's visits. During that time, he and I became good friends because we spent practically every waking moment of the day together. We watched a ton of his favorite movies, went on nice walks through the neighborhood, and shot BB guns in the backyard, until sadly, after five months, he passed away from liver cancer. So, he lived three months longer than what the doctors had expected.

It was at that point when I realized what that dream from my mother months prior had meant. It meant that it was time for me to go on a mission to first change the misfortunes of my own health then help others do the same. I'm 5'2" and weighed in at approximately 185 pounds; I was about 60 pounds overweight. My Body Mass Index (BMI) had climbed to the point where I was now considered obese, along with having both prediabetes and heart disease. During this time, I had no idea what being healthy really looked like, because I hadn't been healthy for quite some time. For most of my adult life, my cholesterol had always been moderately high because I enjoyed the taste of food, especially during the holidays. Thanksgiving was always my favorite time because I got to visit with family and eat a lot of food. I would often have competitions with my nephews just to see who could eat the most turkey, pork roast, candied yams, macaroni and cheese, neck bones, cornbread, and sweet potato pies.

But all of that changed after the passing of my mother. I started doing extensive research into sickness and disease, because I wanted to know why she had passed away so suddenly. I wanted to know exactly what causes a heart attack and where they come from. I wanted to know what cancer was and where it came from. I literally turned myself into a "mad scientist" looking for these answers. So, the more research I conducted, the more I kept getting pointed back to the food. But what was it about the food that I needed to know? Well, as you will find out in Chapter 3, food can either be the slowest poison or the best form of medicine. So, in 2021, I went back to school, and I've since become a Certified Holistic Nutritionist with a specialty in Plant-Based Medicine for disease prevention.

Had someone told me about plant-based nutrition or being vegan prior to tragically losing my loved ones, I would have probably *laughed* in their face, because there was no way in hell that I was ever giving up my double cheeseburgers with extra pickles and a small fry for fruits and vegetables. Nevertheless, I followed the research and the science, but more importantly, I followed The Laws of Nature. In 2021, I went from the worst shape of my life to the best shape of my life in a matter of 10 months, down from 185 to 115 pounds. I was no longer a prediabetic, and I was given only a 3% chance of having a heart attack over the next 10 years versus the grim diagnosis that I had received almost one year prior. I'm now back to my high school weight and for a guy in his mid-40s, *high school* was a very long time ago. In the coming chapters of this book, I will shed light onto everything I've learned during my own health struggles, as well as the things I've applied to totally transform my health.

I discovered that if you can understand how nature truly works, then you'll understand how most of these common diseases are formed within the human body. Each chapter will begin with either an analogy or a story that I've either lived or experienced in some way. My teaching style and delivery may come across as a bit unorthodox, so if you're reading something that may seem a bit wacky, or weird, just know that it will have a meaning and will make perfect sense by the end of the chapter. This book will probably challenge a lot of your beliefs, but in the end, who are *we* to argue with "*Mother Nature*?" After reading this book you will be armed with the same tools and knowledge that I've used and applied to totally transform my health. It is my hope to take you on a thrill ride and on a journey into the mind of a "mad scientist," so let's dive in!

Chapter 1

THE LAWS OF NATURE

Whether you're looking to lose weight and keep it off or if you're trying to heal your body from some type of chronic disease or condition, you'll first need to understand and really grasp the concept of healing the body naturally through the power of nature and plant-based nutrition. But to understand true healing, you must first and foremost understand life on planet earth: the place we all call home.

The earth was created a very, very long time ago and more specifically it was created over 2.5 billion years ago, well before you and I were born. So, regardless of your religious background or faith, would you agree with me that we all have a creator? Or would you agree to there being some form of a higher power? From here on, I will refer to that "higher power" as "Mother Nature," so even if you believe in the Big Bang Theory, you will still have a creator. And when the creator created this planet, there was also a very specific and special diet created. A special diet was created for each of the living species who inhabit the earth, because *Mother Nature* is perfect in her design, and she does not make mistakes. So, let's dive into it.

When it comes to food and what you should be eating, *Mother Nature* has already taken most of the guesswork out of it based on three special diets. For the most part, all life on earth will fall into one of three categories and those categories are herbivore, carnivore, and omnivore. Our anatomy and genetic makeup will tell us exactly what we should be eating, and here's what I mean by that.

Herbivore, Carnivore, Omnivore

Herbivore

An organism that only feeds on plants, herbivores can range in size from tiny insects all the way up to huge elephants. Everything about an herbivore says that it is designed to eat plant material from nature. That includes everything from their teeth, fingers and toes, hooves, digestive systems, saliva, jar structure, how fast they can run, and even down to their gut bacteria. Here are some examples of herbivores: horses, cows, giraffes, deer, antelope, gorillas, sheep, goats, rabbits, squirrels, mice, elephants, camels, zebras, and many more!

But what is it about an herbivore that makes them want to eat vegetation or plants? The answer is "simple" and it's in their anatomy. Nature has already decided this for them, so it's instinctual for them to gravitate towards plants, because that's how *Mother Nature* has designed them.

Example 1:
The teeth of herbivores are flat because they are designed to move in a grinding/side to side/circular motion, also known as chewing. The next time you see a cow or deer, have a look at how they're *chewing* their food, and look at how flat their teeth are.

Example 2:
Herbivores will usually have fingers or hooves; fingers are generally used for picking up or grasping things, while hooves, on the other hand, help these animals walk and run on hard surfaces. In animals like horses and antelope, hooves are an adaptation for fast running and lend the animal both speed and endurance. This is the reason you'll only see horses at the Kentucky Derby, because of how incredibly fast these animals can run. The sharp hooves of some of these animals are used for defense to fight off hungry carnivores, which we'll talk about next.

Example 3:

The digestive system of an herbivore is extremely long; it is roughly 3 times the length of a carnivore's digestive system. Why is that? It's because nature has specifically designed their long digestive systems for the digestion of plant matter. Plants have a lot of nutrients including vitamins, minerals, and phytonutrients (Phyto=nutrients found only in plants for disease prevention). So, it takes their bodies a lot longer to properly absorb all the nutrients from the plants.

Carnivores

An animal or organism that feeds primarily on flesh, specifically *raw flesh,* are also known as meat eaters. They were designed by *Mother Nature* herself to specifically eat other animals. The instinct of a carnivore is to chase, catch, and devour its prey while it's still alive. They have no regard for the life of its prey, only to eat it. A carnivore does not care if it's consuming a newborn baby monkey or a full-grown elephant. The idea is to eat the raw flesh of its prey by any means necessary. After they consume the flesh, they don't feel bad about it, because that's what nature designed them to do.

Here are some examples of carnivores: lions, tigers, alligators, leopards, sharks, cheetahs, hyenas, wild dogs, wolves, and even spiders.

Example 1:

Carnivores, unlike herbivores, have different jaw structures; their jaws are designed to move in only two directions, and that's up and down. This is because they have sharp teeth made for piercing through the flesh of their prey. I grew up in Florida, so if you've ever watched a Florida Gators football game, you'll notice the crowd is doing what's called *"The Chomp."* The crowd will cheer for a big play with an up and down motion using their arms, signifying an alligator eating its prey. The reason the fans do this is because they are aware of alligators being known carnivores, and that is how carnivores devour their food. They don't chew their food; they rip the flesh from the bones of their prey and eat it while it's *still* alive. At times, they can be flat out unmerciful! So, growing up in Florida I knew never to play next to a pond or lake, because there could be a very good chance of there being a hungry alligator lying just below the surface of the water.

Example 2:

Carnivores have claws instead of fingers. Claws are used to catch and hold their prey, and also used to climb trees at an extremely efficient rate. If you've ever seen a leopard climb a tree, you'll understand exactly what I mean. Once a carnivore catches its prey, there's no need to take it to the stove, oven, or fire pit to be cooked, because it's dinner time right there on the spot! The reason these animals don't need to cook their food is because *Mother Nature* has perfectly designed their digestive tracts to handle *raw flesh*.

Example 3:

Carnivores have much shorter and very simple digestive systems as compared to that of its herbivore counterpart. Have you ever accidentally left a piece of uncooked meat out on the counter for a couple of days? If you have, then you can pretty much guarantee that when you came back the meat would be rotting and decaying with a very foul odor. Carnivores eat raw flesh. *Mother Nature* knows this, because that's how she designed them. So, she specifically designed their digestive systems to be short and simple to quickly eliminate the rotting flesh of the other animals they've been eating. So, it doesn't matter if meat is left out on the counter for days or if it's inside the digestive tract of a living organism, it's still going to rot! I live in Texas, so I drive by lots of cow pastures almost daily. It would be the weirdest thing I have ever seen if one day I passed by those same pastures, and I saw cows (herbivores) eating chunks of meat like carnivores instead of the nice green grasses. I'm pretty sure seeing such an image would probably blow your mind too, but the reason you'd never see something like that is because *Mother Nature* is perfect in her design, and she doesn't make mistakes.

Omnivores

Animals that can eat both plants and the "raw flesh" of other animals are omnivores. *True* omnivores don't need to take their food to the stovetop, oven, or fire pit. They would prefer to dine right there on the spot. Some examples of omnivores include bears, pigs, crawfish, baboons, dogs, raccoons, ostriches, warthogs, and many more. Most of the literature and advertising on television says that human beings are omnivores. If that's the case then ask yourself why are humans the only omnivores that must take the *raw flesh* of the other animals they eat to the oven, stovetop, or firepit? These are the questions I had to ask myself when I decided to go on a vegan journey to change the fortunes of my health. I needed to take a deep dive into health and wellness, because like I mentioned in the introductory chapter, I had no intentions of ever giving up my double cheeseburgers with extra pickles and a small fry. So, I'll let you decide for yourself which category you believe humans belong in once you finish this chapter.

Life at Sea

As I mentioned earlier, I spent over a decade in the US Navy on various battleships touring the world and serving my country. And in that time, I saw about as much water and sea life that you could possibly ever want to imagine. Basically, I've seen a lot of water in my years of life on this planet. With that, the next question I had to ask myself was "can I still eat fish if I go vegan???" I had always heard that we as humans need to get our Omega-3 fatty acids, which is an *essential nutrient* from a fish source. This nutrient is needed for optimal brain and heart health, so we are told to get it from sources like salmon, mackerel, oysters, caviar, and other seafood. So, then the question became, "If human beings can't breathe underwater without man-made scuba gear, and if it's almost impossible to catch a fish naturally with my bare hands, why the hell would *Mother Nature* put this essential nutrient below the surface of the water if she knew that I couldn't breathe under there?" I thought to myself, "what type of mother would do that?" Heck! I was almost tempted to call (CPS) Child Protective Services, for the sake of poor parenting, BUT I digress!

In actual reality, Omega-3 fatty acids come from the seaweed or algae found in the oceans, and the process goes something like this... The fish don't naturally produce this essential nutrient. Once a fish in the ocean eats the seaweed or algae, which provides the natural Omega-3 to the fish, it is then infused within the flesh of the fish. Once we catch and consume the fish, now we have the Omega-3. It's like a high-stakes game of tag, only this game involves your health. Our oceans are heavily polluted with all types of disease-causing toxins, so you may want to ask yourself, "is consuming seafood to get your Omega-3 fatty acids really the best option or is there an alternative?"

I say cut out the middleman and go straight for an algae or seaweed supplement. There are also many plant-based sources like chia seeds, flax seeds, walnuts, hemp seeds, and Brussels sprouts. I'd also like to mention that an ocean filled with fish is great for the overall health of our planet. As I mentioned earlier *Mother Nature* doesn't make mistakes, there is a reason human beings can't breathe underwater. To put it simply, it's because nature did not design us that way. So again, I'll let you make your own determination as to whether human beings are designed to eat fish.

Human Baby vs. Lion Cub Analogy

If you have children, you'll know exactly what I mean when I say "The Terrible Twos." Imagine if you took a two-year-old human baby and placed them in the playpen for a couple of hours because you had chores to do. Let's face it, we all have things to do around the house, whether we like it or not! In this analogy, I'm not deciding for you: I'll let you come to your own conclusions.

Scenario 1: A Two-Year-Old Human Baby:

You leave for a couple of hours, and to keep the baby occupied you leave an apple, and a live bunny rabbit in the playpen with the baby. When you returned two hours later, which one would the baby have eaten, and which one would the baby have played with? The apple or the live bunny rabbit?

Scenario 2: A Two-Year-Old Lion Cub:

Now, let's rewind that exact same scenario, but this time we'll replace the two-year-old human baby with a two-year-old lion cub. We would still have the same apple and the *live* bunny rabbit in the playpen. But this time, when you returned two hours later, which one would the lion cub have eaten, and which one would the lion cub have played with? Would you expect the live bunny rabbit to still be alive or would you expect the worst?

Remember, I'm not deciding for you, but my guess is that in scenario 1, the two-year-old human baby would have eaten the apple and would have played with the bunny rabbit. In scenario 2, the lion cub would have eaten the live bunny rabbit and would have played with the apple. Wait, on second thought...lions don't play with apples! So, I'm sure the apple would still be there upon your return. I say all of this to say that *Mother Nature* doesn't make mistakes. Two-year-old babies don't comprehend all that well, but one thing they do understand is how to follow their nature. It would probably be the weirdest scenario in the world if you came back two hours later to find out the human baby has eaten the live bunny rabbit and has played with the apple. The first thing you'd probably say is "oh my goodness! That baby is going to get sick!"

Well, fast forward throughout the lifespan of a human and then ask yourself, "how many people do you know that have either passed away from sickness or they are suffering from some type of disease?"

Here's the link: we as humans are still eating that live bunny rabbit, but the only difference is we are now just seasoning and cooking the bunny rabbit on the stovetop, in an oven, or on a fire pit! And as I just mentioned, there's a very good chance that you'll probably "*get sick!*" In the next chapter, we'll dig a little bit deeper into where most sickness and diseases come from and how they are formed within the body.

Chapter 2

WHY ARE WE SO SICK?

The Werewolf Gene Analogy

Growing up as a kid my mother would love to watch television shows involving werewolves and vampires (all fictional of course). But for this example, I want to focus on the werewolf gene. In these television shows, there are two ways to become a full-blown werewolf, and trust me, being a werewolf is a *very* extreme thing to become. That means you would be running around through the woods at night as a man or she-wolf, while howling at the moon and chasing your prey. So, it's safe to say that you probably would not want to be a werewolf. The two ways to become a werewolf are: being born with the gene or if another werewolf bites you.

If you're born with the werewolf gene, it doesn't necessarily mean anything until you've triggered the *curse*. The curse is triggered by doing something very extreme, and I hate to say this, but you become a werewolf by taking someone's life caused by either an accident or on purpose. It is at that point when the curse is triggered, and you have now become a full-blown werewolf howling at the full moon, chasing, and eating the *raw flesh* from the bones of your prey just like a *true* carnivore! But had you not triggered the curse, you would have simply lived your life as a normal everyday person. That was a very extreme analogy to give, but by the end of this chapter you'll understand why becoming a werewolf is such an extreme thing to become. As you get to know me, you'll understand how much I love using analogies in my teachings. It's something I picked up during my years as an instructor at the US Naval Academy.

Diesel vs. Unleaded Fuel

According to a recent study conducted by the National Health Interview Survey published in 2018, the latest estimates show more than 52 percent of adults in the United States have at least one chronic condition. Another 27 percent of the American population has two or more chronic conditions with millions of others who haven't even been diagnosed yet. According to the survey these are the top 10 diseases or conditions: arthritis, cancer, COPD, heart disease, asthma, diabetes, hepatitis, hypertension, strokes, and kidney disease. These are just to name a few, but these are the top conditions that make up the

52 percent. Those are staggering numbers, so that means more than half of the adults in America have some type of chronic disease or condition, but the question is why? Why is it that more than half of the American population suffers from either a chronic disease or an illness? The answer lies within the fuel source that we choose to run on. Our fuel source determines if our body is going to express health or if it's going to express a sickness or a disease. There are many other factors within our environments that can also contribute to a disease, but most disease development and its progression is determined by your fuel source. There are two types of fuel sources. Allow me to explain what I mean by your fuel source.

Diesel Fuel

Diesel fuel makes up 90% of the Standard American Diet (S.A.D.). It's a hard pill to swallow, but most of us are filling up on the wrong fuel source, and it's causing the cells within our bodies to go haywire. Most of us probably grew up on diesel fuel, as I know I certainly did! Diesel fuel is the main contributor for 70% of the American population being either overweight or obese.

Diesel fuel:
60% Processed foods
30% Animal products
10% Fruits, veggies, herbs, and spices

Processed Foods

This means it's similar to food, but it's not actually food. It's food-like, but it's not actually real food! To break it down even further, it means once a human being has gotten their hands on it, to shape or manufacture it in any way, or if it's been taken out of its natural plant state and turned into something that your grandmother wouldn't recognize, then it would be considered processed. Most of these products are engineered in a laboratory to achieve a desired texture or taste, and they are specifically designed to keep you coming back for more. On the other hand, there are some minimally processed foods that can be very beneficial for your health, while other things like *ultra-processed foods* can be very harmful and detrimental to your health. Let me explain the difference between the various types of processed foods. According to www.FoodIndustry.com from an article published in November of 2018, the article says there are four categories of processed foods, and they are:

1. **Unprocessed or minimally processed**
2. **Processed culinary ingredients**
3. **Processed foods**
4. **Heavily or ultra-processed food**

That all sounds a bit confusing, so I like viewing it a little differently. I've grouped them into four of my own categories just to give you an easier understanding as to what we're consuming when we eat "*processed foods*."

Minimally Processed Plant Food

Foods that are closest to nature, meaning the food is harvested directly from the source with minimal to no alterations, are also known as whole food. The truth of the matter is that most of the foods we eat in today's world must go through some level of processing. Foods such as sliced fruits and vegetables, bagged salads, chopped leafy greens, smoothies, canned beans, and roasted nuts are all examples of minimally processed foods. So again, there are processed foods that are beneficial for our health. The problems begin when we start upping the ante by consuming extremely refined processed foods. The next three categories have little to no health benefits for the human body, as they are the truest definition of *diesel fuel*.

Ultra-Processed Sweetened Beverages

These beverages have little to no nutritional value and they contain high levels of artificial sugars and ingredients. The label may even state that it's an all-natural product that's loaded with vitamins, minerals, antioxidants, and that they may have little to no calories. These beverages are mass produced at high levels of efficiency and are designed to stay stashed away on the shelf at your local supermarket for months on end. Things like sports drinks, most of the store-bought pre-workout formulas, both diet and regular sodas, beer, sweet teas, fruit punch, and energy drinks are some examples of ultra-processed sweetened beverages. They often come in many different flavors designed to mimic the taste of an actual plant. You've seen them on the shelves; flavors like strawberry, grape, watermelon, and orange just to name a few.

Ultra-Processed Food

According to the research, ultra-processed foods should be avoided at all costs. In 2018, a report in *The British Medical Journal* uncovered a link between ultra-processed foods and an increased risk for cancer. Some newer studies say eating even small amounts of processed microwaved tv dinners, fast-food nuggets, or bags of chips a few times a week has been associated with major health drawbacks.

Ultra-processed foods are products that use additives such as sweeteners, emulsifiers, preservatives, artificial colors, and flavors. They're often high in calories, refined sugars, fat, and sodium. Here's a good way to easily identify ultra-processed foods. Have a look at the nutritional label on the back—if you see an entire laundry list full of unpronounceable or unrecognizable ingredients, there's a very good chance that it's ultra-processed. As I mentioned earlier, "If your grandmother wouldn't recognize it, then it's probably best to put it back on the shelf." Let me give you some examples of these health harming foods: Sweetened breakfast cereals like Captain Crunch™, cakes, cookies, crackers, pizza, candy, tv dinners, white sugar, refined white flour, most breads, donuts, ramen instant noodles, and fake vegan burgers or patties. These products are made from very low levels of *real* plant ingredients, and they have little to no nutritional value products like Beyond™ and Impossible™ Burgers and many others.

We also call them "refined foods" meaning the food has gone through a refining process to remove most, and if not all, of the naturally reoccurring plant nutrients and fibers. This is done to preserve the shelf life of a particular product. Have you ever noticed an unopened box of cereal can stay stored on the shelf for months on end without going stale? If you ever left an actual live plant on a shelf for months without giving it any TLC, it wouldn't survive because plants need soil, sunlight, and water to flourish. In other words, plants are alive, so in turn they give us life.

Processed Animal Products

Whether it's something obvious such as meat, or perhaps a surprising case such as wine, many of the goods and foods we buy contain ingredients that fall under the category of "animal products" or "animal by-products." According to the Animal and Plant Health Inspection Service (APHIS), a division formed by the U.S. Department of Agriculture (USDA) in 1972, animal products are materials derived from the body of an animal.

The list of specific parts and substances include:

- Skin
- Meat
- Fat
- Organs
- Blood
- Milk
- Fish
- Eggs
- Hair
- Bones
- Hooves
- Jell-O (a protein derived from the skin and bones of certain animals)
- Rennet: (the stomach contents of an unweaned hooved animal just prior to digestion, most likely from a calf) it has traditionally been used to separate milk into solid curds and liquid, in other words, it's used to make cheese (more on this later)

- Gelatin (usually comes from collagen in various animal body parts)

All meat that has been smoked, salted, cured, dried, or canned is considered processed. Things like sausages, hot dogs, salami, ham, deli meats, canned tuna, beef jerky, and cured bacon are processed. Processed meat has consistently been linked with having harmful effects on human health. This is something that most health-conscious people have been aware of for many decades. Heck, I sure wish this was something that I had known in my younger years, because I used to eat these products like they were going out of style. Our taste buds really love the taste of these highly processed foods, so they are designed with taste in mind! But even though our taste buds may love it, our body absolutely hates it!

In 2015, based on data from over 800 studies, The World Health Organization (WHO) classified processed meat as a Group 1 carcinogen. This means there is enough evidence to conclude that it can cause cancer in humans. The problem with most processed foods is they have little to no nutritional value for that of human physiology. Most of the essential vitamins, nutrients, and fibers have been stripped away during the refining process, and other preservatives have been added to create structure, texture, flavor, and to add shelf life to the product. The processed food industry is well aware of this, but to them it's all about the profit, not human health, because let's face it: *money* makes the world go around!

Let's switch gears a bit and discuss the other fuel source.

Unleaded

Based on human anatomy, there is no denying that we are *true* plant eaters (herbivores). We have very similar and long digestive systems just like most of the herbivores mentioned in Chapter 1. With that being said, the optimal fuel source designed by *Mother Nature* herself is for human beings to run on plants and vegetation. Everything about human anatomy says that we are plant eaters, as you will hear me mention several times throughout this book. *Mother Nature* does not make mistakes. Earth, as we know it, is the only planet capable of supporting and sustaining various life forms, from the countless animal species to some of the most complex ecosystems like the rainforests, which were designed to keep the earth cool just like your home's air conditioning unit. She is perfect in her design!

Unleaded fuel is the opposite of diesel fuel.

Unleaded:
90% = fruits, vegetables, whole grains, legumes (beans) nuts, seeds, herbs, and spices
10% = processed junk food or animal products

Unleaded fuel has minimal to no processing, and as I mentioned earlier, pretty much all the food in today's world is processed in some shape, form, or fashion. But the key is to eat as closely to nature as possible by consuming whole plant foods. Here are some examples of minimal to no processed whole plant foods: apples, oranges, kale, spinach, carrots, beets, onions, lemons, limes, beans, avocados, peppers, whole grains like quinoa, brown rice, oats, bulgur wheat, and the list goes on and on. To make it even easier to understand, these are the foods primarily found in the produce section at your local grocery store.

These foods give your body life. As I mentioned earlier, plants need three things to sustain themselves: nutrient rich soil, light, and water. When we consume life-giving foods at least 90% of the time, magical things will start to happen within our cells. I'm not saying that you have to be like me by going 100% vegan or plant-based, but I am saying to fill up on an unleaded fuel source *most* of the time. *Especially* if you're trying to heal your body from a condition like Type 2 Diabetes or some other ailment, then watch how your body transforms itself!

Fad Diets

Fad diets are plans sold as the best and fastest approach for losing weight. Yet, some of these diets involve eliminating foods that contain the necessary nutrients your body needs to maintain good health. Throughout my life, I've tried many of these fad diets in hopes of losing weight quickly. Here are a couple examples of fad diets; Ketogenic, Atkins, The South Beach Diet, Nutrisystem™, Weight Watchers™, The Grapefruit Diet, Paleo, The DASH diet, and that's just to name a few, but there are many more. These diets are dangerous because they lack the true nutrients needed to maintain good health. As Rip Esselstyn from the Plantstrong podcast would say, these diets are filled with C.R.A.P. (Calorie Rich And Processed) and mostly artificial ingredients.

Another way of remembering this acronym is:

- C-Carbonated Junk
- R-Refined Sugars
- A-Artificial Stuff
- P-Processed Foods

Our body does not recognize the artificial ingredients found in most of these diets. This in turn sends the wrong signals to the trillions of cells within the body, which can cause them to do weird and funky stuff. Think of your body like a credit card transaction: we can charge a bunch of C.R.A.P. in our youth i.e... tons of diesel fuel, but I don't care how many years have gone by, that credit card company will still track you down to get their money from you even if you've forgotten about it. So, in essence you can charge all the bad junk food today, but tomorrow it will be time to pay up. And paying up is defined as going into the hospital or doctor's office to get the latest and greatest prescription, or by having some expensive but totally avoidable surgery to alleviate our symptoms. Chronic inflammation is the main driver for the development of a chronic disease; it's your body's way of telling you to start toning down the diesel fuel, but we hardly ever listen to our bodies. When we don't listen, that chronic inflammation can and will turn into a chronic disease or a condition.

The Disease Delusion

Did you know that 90-95% of all disease is preventable? As I mentioned at the start of this chapter, triggering the *werewolf curse* is totally extreme, but avoidable, unless you do something totally extreme to trigger the curse. Think of it like this, if you go to the gas station and you accidentally fill your car up with diesel fuel instead of the optimal fuel source of petrol (unleaded fuel), what do you think would happen to your car? An old coworker of mine told me a story about how his 17-year-old daughter borrowed the family van to go visit with a friend, but when she brought the van back it was shaking like a leaf. His daughter didn't know the difference between diesel and the unleaded fuel, so she proceeded to fill the van with diesel fuel. To make a long story short, he told me that he had to spend thousands of dollars to get the van's engine repaired. But the crazy thing is after getting the engine fixed, the van still runs, but it runs like trash! The moral of that story is had his daughter simply filled up with the unleaded fuel, which was the correct fuel source for the van, it would have saved him so much time and money, and the family's van would still be running like a champ!

Well, it's the same thing for the human body: if you fill up with diesel fuel most of the time, your body will start to break down, and it will eventually start to run like trash because it's the wrong fuel source for human anatomy. But if you flip things by filling up on the correct fuel source (aka unleaded) most of the time which are fruits, veggies, legumes, whole grains, nuts, and seeds, you'll start to notice positive changes in your health. Unlike the car engine, the human body is designed to repair itself, so all you have to do is give it the time and the correct fuel it needs to properly work its magic. So, in other words, you only have a 5-10% chance of triggering a disease and becoming a werewolf. But, most of us will trigger the disease curse at some point in our lives by doing something very extreme, and the extreme thing that most humans do is fill up on diesel fuel 90% of the time. Again, there are other factors within our environments that can contribute to a disease. But 9 times out of 10, it is your fuel source and lifestyle that has caused you to become a full-blown werewolf, now howling at the moon while chasing your prey through the woods at night, *not* family genetics!

Identical Twins Analogy

I grew up with a set of identical twins, so I very much understand the dynamic between the two, and as it also turns out, twins share identical genes. So, for this example, let's say these twins have a family history of Type 2 Diabetes. But twin A grew up consuming only unleaded fuel and has continued this way of eating for his or her entire life. Twin B, on the other hand, grew up consuming diesel fuel and has continued eating this way throughout his or her entire life. When they turn 30 years old, twin B has become extremely overweight and has just been diagnosed with the family curse of Type 2 Diabetes. While twin A, on the other hand, is well within a healthy body weight and has no signs of Type 2 Diabetes. Why? Doesn't the diabetes curse run in their family? Shouldn't both twins trigger the diabetes curse? Why is it that twin A is very healthy with no signs of the disease, but twin B has the disease? The answer is simple, twin A never triggered the diabetes curse because he or she filled up on unleaded fuel the entire time. Twin B did the total opposite and chose to fill up on diesel fuel the entire time, which caused his or her cells to go haywire, and in turn triggering the disease. So, for me the answer as to "why are we SO sick?" lies directly in front of you, and it's the food, it's the food, it's the food!

Chapter 3

MEDICINE ISN'T HEALTHCARE, FOOD IS HEALTHCARE

"*Mother Nature*" can destroy life, but she can also give you a second chance at life! In August of 2017, I married my wife with the intention of living our happily ever after, but nature had other plans for us. I live in Texas, so if you've watched the news in recent years, you've probably heard of Hurricane Harvey... Shortly after returning home from our honeymoon, Hurricane Harvey came knocking at our front door; we didn't even have a chance to really put away our wedding gifts. So, when the waters from the storm began to rise, and as I'm watching some of my lifelong work and credentials get destroyed by the flood waters, and three of my vehicles getting destroyed, ALL I could do was cry! And as I'm watching my home get destroyed all I could do was continue to cry. It got to the point where the authorities had to send in boats to rescue some of my neighbors. I called my insurance company and I cried to them too. I cried to anyone who would listen, but it didn't matter who I cried to or how much I cried, because an act of nature does *not* care! So again, she can destroy your life, but she can also give "you" a second chance at LIFE! By the end of this chapter, you'll understand what I mean by giving "you" life.

Medicine Has Its Place, but Only if It's Needed

Years ago when my wife and I first met, we went on a seven-day cruise to the Caribbean. I distinctly remember being taught a very specific lesson by one of the group excursion tour guides. Someone from our tour group raised their hand and asked him a question. "Mr. Tour guide," they said, "where or how do you get your medicine here?" He replied, "from the land." She replied with a follow-up question: "well what about when you get diseases?" He replied, "all the medicine we need is right here within this land," he continued to say, "If we get sick, we go to the land, grab the natural plants, mix them together with another plant and that's *how* we get our medicine!" And finally, he replied, "but no one really gets sick here." On another note, he did show us this really cool trick for how to eat ants without getting stung. I told him, "No disrespect brother, but I'll pass on the ants!" I really didn't understand the gravity of that lesson until years later when my own health challenges began.

As I mentioned earlier, in late 2020, I was diagnosed with both prediabetes and heart disease at the very same doctor's visit. And after my bloodwork comes back with extremely high cholesterol numbers, my doctor has one of the nurses give me a call to prescribe a statin. They tell me that I also have symptoms of angina. "The technical term for angina (an-JIE-nuh or AN-juh-nuh) is a type of chest pain caused by reduced blood flow to the heart. Angina is a symptom of coronary artery disease; it's also called *angina pectoris*. When I heard this devastating news, I immediately experienced a low moment because I took pride in the fact that up until this point, I had never been prescribed long-term medication.

Sure, I'd pop a Motrin or Ibuprofen if I ever had a headache, or I'd use an over-the-counter antacid if I were ever having indigestion or something like that, but nothing serious. I'd take the meds for a day or two just until the headache symptoms went away or if my tummy started feeling better. Then I'd throw the Motrin bottle to the back of the medicine cabinet until the next time I needed it. But now, I had to face the reality of being diagnosed with a heart condition, all while thinking about how my mother had just passed away months prior from a heart attack! So, this was a wake-up call for me. The technical term I gave you was for the Latin word *"Angina Pectoris,"* meaning to have pain in your chest. Allow me to paint the picture of what it feels like to have this condition. It's essentially an early warning sign that any day could be your last. It meant that if I didn't stop eating my double cheeseburgers with extra pickles, small fries, pork chops, sour gummy worms, Taco Bell™, buffalo wings, and washing it all down with a Mountain Dew™. That I was going to be having a heart attack at any time!

Sometimes I could just be hanging out on my sofa while watching a football game and I would feel excruciating pain in my chest. But the pain didn't stop there, it would often travel down my left arm and sometimes it would get so bad that it would drop me to my knees. The only thing that helped was just sitting down and taking really slow, deep breaths for a few minutes until the pain subsided. Walking up and down stairs became a challenge, because I would often have shortness of breath, especially in places with higher altitudes like Colorado. Bending over to tie my shoes also became quite the challenge, because doing that would often trigger a response in my chest. Take it from me, having this condition is no walk in the park, as it can lead to some devastating consequences! So, the question I had to ask myself was "what am I going to do about it?" Because having a heart attack was very likely in my near future, was I going to suffer the inevitable or was I going to do something about it? Was I going to take the newly prescribed statin medication from my doctor or was I going to do something different?

I started racking my brain like *crazy* to come up with a solution. As I mentioned, up until this diagnosis I had taken pride in living a medication-free life. But it was at this moment when I remembered the lesson taught to my excursion group. I thought back to what the tour guide said, and I quote, "we don't get our medicine from the local grocery store, we get our medication from the land." And "no one hardly ever gets sick here, but if someone did get sick, we'd go out into the bushes, grab the plants we needed. Mix the plants together into some type of concoction, drink or eat it, then we would just *let* nature take its course." Some people may call it an epiphany, but I knew what I had to do. I received the news in December of 2020 about my condition, so on January 1 of 2021, I decided that enough was enough, and I decided to live a Whole-Foods, Plant-Based Vegan Lifestyle.

I decided that I was going to give it 100%. So, I started using the lessons taught to us on that cruise excursion. I started experimenting on myself with only plants, I eliminated processed foods and animal products (diesel fuel) from my diet, and within a span of 10 months I had lost about 65 pounds. I went from having a *dad bod*, prediabetes, and a heart condition, to a fit and energetic kid, because I'm now back to my high school weight, which I hadn't seen in over a quarter of a century. So, I went back to the doctor and my new bloodwork came back with no signs of prediabetes, my total cholesterol had dropped by nearly 100 points, and I was given only a 3% chance of having a heart attack within the next 10 years. I did this without taking any of the prescribed statins or medications from my doctor. Instead, I decided to do what the tour guide from the excursion group taught me, and that was "to just *let* nature take its course."

The point of that story was to educate you on the power of *nature*. What I've discovered is that prescription medication does have its place within our society, but *nature* will always reign supreme! If taking prescription medicine is needed at the time, I encourage you to listen to your doctor. But I like to compare taking prescription medications and over the counter drugs to the 4x100 Track and Field relay at the Olympics. The relay has four participants. Each participant must run a short 100 meters, then they hand the baton off to the next leg of the race until it reaches the anchor; the anchor grabs the baton and takes it all the way to the finish line. Your body operates the same way: medication is ok for a short period of time if it's needed, but just like in the 4x100 relay, it should be for a very short period. My stance is this:

Mother Nature is perfect and everything that we need, she supplies!

Having great health and getting the proper nutrition is what nature intended. So, if you start with the basics of proper nutrition, the rest will take care of itself. All that is required of you is to give your body the proper fuel that it needs. Plants come directly from nature, and just like when Hurricane Harvey came through and destroyed my home, there wasn't anything I could do to stop the rising flood waters from destroying our home, because that was an act of nature! It works the exact same way with plants, as they also come from nature. So, just like I mentioned at the start of this chapter, *"Mother Nature"* can destroy your life, but she can also give you a second chance at life.

I was given a second chance at life so that I could write this book to let you know that *you* can also have a second chance at life. The Centers for Disease Control and Prevention (CDC) concluded in a study from 2020 saying that heart disease is responsible for 1 in 4 deaths in the US. That equates to one person dying every 34 seconds from this condition-- making it the leading cause of death nationwide. I encourage you to not become part of this ugly statistic! Start making lifestyle changes towards regaining your health *today*. Don't wait until tomorrow, because heart attacks can be swift, they can be sudden, and they can be devastating!

Here are some of my own sets of philosophies when it comes to naturally regaining your health:

1. First, you must take care of yourself because you cannot help others if your health is also suffering. You do this by using nature as your weapon, because there is no force more powerful than nature itself. Plants are from nature, so use them to your advantage.

2. If it came from a plant, eat it! But if it was manufactured by man, then there is a very good chance that you should probably put it back on the shelf.

3. The old adage of eating an apple a day to keep the doctor away is great, but the day is longer than you may think, so make time for your health and eat more plants!

Dr. Joel Fuhrman said it best in his book published in 2011 called *Super Immunity* when he said: "Medicines cannot drug away the cellular defects that develop in response to improper nutrition throughout life."

But the philosophy that really drives home this point comes from Michael Pollan when he said in his book titled *In Defense of Food* published in January of 2008: "Eat food, not too much, mostly plants." We'll dig a little deeper into this philosophy in the next chapter.

Last, but certainly not least, there is a famous quote by Hippocrates that you've probably heard, and it says "Let food be thy medicine, and let medicine be thy food." To simplify that, it means to eat the natural whole plant foods for which nature has perfectly designed for your body. And nature will take that baton (4x100 relay) all the way to the finish line. It means using a prescription medication to alleviate your short-term symptoms is ok, but *true* medicine is perfectly packaged within the natural plants for which was given to us by *Mother Nature* herself.

Chapter 4

WEIGHT LOSS 101

Why Can't I Keep the Weight Off?

That's probably a question most of us have asked ourselves countless times over the years. I know I surely have! I would ask myself, "why did I just lose a bunch of weight only to gain it back within six months or so?" At my heaviest, I had gotten up to 185 pounds. For a gentleman who stands five feet, two inches tall, that is a lot of extra weight! But up until reaching this all-time high, I had tried pretty much everything that you could ever imagine to lose the weight and keep it off. Some things would work for a little while. I'd lose a few pounds, then the second I let my guard down, boom! The weight would come roaring back. This was my journey for most of my adult life, so when I first started my health and weight loss journey, I had absolutely NO idea what I was doing. If you're reading this book, then there's probably a very good chance that you and I share similar weight loss journeys and stories.

- I tried pretty much all the fad and yo-yo diets on the market...
- I exercised both day and night...
- I counted millions of calories...
- I weighed my food...
- I counted macronutrients...
- Intermittent fasting...
- Portion-controlled diets...
- I tried Nutrisystem (twice)

When I look back at it, I've realized that I was doing basically everything wrong...What I was doing is called "Yo-Yo Dieting."

Microwave vs. Oven Approach

The clinical term for yo-yo dieting is called "weight cycling," which means gaining weight unintentionally and "dieting" in response, losing the weight then regaining the weight, then you go on another weight loss journey, only to gain it back again! In simple terms, it means your weight is going up and down like a yo-yo. The cycle repeats itself year after year and decade after decade. Why?? To get a better handle on finding the answer to this common problem of "yo-yo dieting," I remembered a lesson taught to me by my grandmother when I was a child. She said, "Son, for your food to taste great and to get the desired texture, I should use the oven instead of the microwave." She emphasized the point of a slower, more natural way of cooking instead of the quick and fast ways of the microwave. Now, as an adult, I remembered the lessons she taught me, and I've used those lessons to keep the weight off. I learned that our bodies work the exact same way as the *oven* and *microwave.*

Fad and yo-yo diets are like using the microwave approach, meaning they are a quick fix to a long-term problem. You may lose some weight, your bloodwork may improve, you may start feeling better, but the second you go back to your normal routine, "guess what?" The weight comes back with a vengeance! Instead of going through this vicious cycle repeatedly, let's use the "oven" approach, which is what I teach to my clients. It means weight loss should be three things: **slow, gradual, and natural**. Once I grasped this concept, it only took approximately five months to lose 45 pounds. I went from being obese to being well within a normal body weight for my height. My shirt size went from an XL to a medium. I was thrilled, but when I looked into the mirror, I knew that I could afford to lose another 20 pounds or so. By the time it was all said and done, I had lost close to 70 pounds. I didn't count a single calorie or macro, nor did I weigh my food on a scale. As a matter of fact, this was the most enjoyable weight loss experience of my life.

Don't Count Your Calories, Instead Eat Real Food

Real food- It basically means eating food that has not been heavily processed. Foods with no artificial additives and foods containing only five or fewer *whole* ingredients. Real food is food that hasn't been artificially created, so that means mostly avoiding ingredients that you cannot pronounce.

Avoid ingredients that you wouldn't cook with at home, and more importantly, it means don't eat foods that your grandmother wouldn't recognize. In simple terms *"real food"* is wholesome and nourishing. It is simple, unprocessed, whole, unrefined food. Real food is pure and unadulterated, sustained yet unchanged by man. Here are some examples of real food, aka Unleaded Fuel.

1. Natural fruits and vegetables

2. Whole Grains (like quinoa, brown rice, corn, whole oats, millet, farro, whole grain breads and pastas, etc....)

3. Nuts and seeds

4. Water and herbal tea

5. Herbs and spices

6. Beans and legumes (black, pinto, navy, kidney, chickpeas, lentils, mung beans and many more)

You may have noticed that I didn't add any animal products, heavily processed junk foods, or sugary drinks to the real food category. That's because this goes back to my explanation of diesel fuel from chapter two. It's simple: diesel fuel has very little to none of the required fiber! Well, now you're probably asking yourself, what exactly is *fiber* and why is it a required nutrient for humans?

Fiber

Fiber is an essential nutrient that can reduce the glycemic index of certain foods and helps keep your blood sugar stable. Fiber has the ability to slow digestion and can reduce blood sugar spikes by between 10 and 20%. This is especially beneficial for stabilizing your blood sugar if you suffer from diabetes. Take fruit for example. Fruit is loaded with natural sugars. So, is it best for a person with Type 2 Diabetes to totally avoid fruit? The answer is "*no,*" eat as much fruit as you'd like, because as I will mention quite often throughout this book, "*Mother Nature*" is perfect in her design. She knows that fruit has tons of sugar, so she specifically designed fruit with fiber in mind. Each piece of fruit that you eat (if eaten in its whole, natural form) will contain the appropriate amounts of fiber to basically cancel out the effects of the sugar.

As you've heard me mention, I was prediabetic before I made the transition to a plant-based vegan lifestyle. During my nearly 70-pound weight loss journey, I ate tons of fruit, and I never once had a problem with extreme blood sugar spikes. Everything was well within a normal tolerance. Fiber is also great for your gut health because it feeds your good gut bacteria and it starves the harmful bacteria. Having great gut health is essential and vital, because having poor gut health can lead to increased risks for many chronic diseases. Poor gut health can lead to conditions like heart disease, diabetes, and some intestinal problems like constipation, IBS and Crohn's disease. Fiber is an essential nutrient only found in *real* plants. Fiber is the nutrient that makes you take regular trips to the bathroom, and it makes your digestive system very happy.

Last but certainly not least, fiber is the messenger between your stomach and brain that tells you to stop eating because you've had enough. It also keeps you feeling fuller for longer. Without the appropriate amounts of fiber in your diet, your brain never receives the signal to stop eating. When we as humans fill up on the wrong fuel source (diesel fuel) 90% of the time, that signal to stop eating never makes it to the appropriate place within our brains. So in turn, we continue to eat and eat until we just can't eat anymore. You may say something like, "I just finished eating an entire meal an hour or two ago, so WHY am I still hungry?" That's because diesel fuel has little to no fiber!

Drop the Idea of Breakfast, Lunch, and Dinner

It sounds far-fetched, but as you will discover in the next chapter, your body has an internal clock called a "circadian rhythm." Eating three square meals a day isn't how nature intended for your cells to operate, because "*true nature*" says to eat when your body is requesting the nutrients. Food is the third most important thing for your survival behind only air and water. Your life is dependent upon the energy source that is generated from inside of your body, and food is the only source of this vital energy. Our body functions by utilizing the energy from the food we eat. Food acts as a fuel source to generate energy for all the living cells within your body. So instead of eating the standard and traditional ways of breakfast, lunch, and dinner, I would suggest listening to your body and the hunger queues it's giving you.

"Eat to live" instead of "living to eat." Eat until you're about 80% full, then push away from the table. As children, we are taught to eat everything on our plates, or else we'd go to bed hungry! So, when we become adults we continue this mentality which can lead to overeating. When your body tells you it's nutrient time, that's when you should eat. Don't eat because the clock says it's breakfast, lunch, or dinner. When we eat three square meals per day of calorically dense foods, our body will store the excess calories in our fat cells until it can figure out what to do with it. So, in essence we are forcing our bodies to take on extra calories that aren't required at the time. This is how the vicious cycle of yo-yo dieting begins. Our weight will go up and down year after year because of these three factors:

1. Eating too much of the wrong fuel (Diesel)

2. Lack of fiber (Diesel fuel has little to no fiber)

3. Eating at the wrong times

Nutrient Dense vs. Calorically Dense Foods

As I mentioned earlier, there is absolutely no need to count calories to regain your health. Counting calories is part of the fad diet culture, but if counting your daily calories works for you, then "hey, I'm on board with it." But, if you're anything like me and you don't have time to constantly keep track of your daily caloric intake with an app or a spreadsheet, then allow me to take you down a different path. When planet earth was created, there were no cell phones, computers, or any other fancy gadgets. If you can understand the difference between nutrient dense vs calorically dense foods, you'll never ever have to worry about counting calories ever again in life, unless it's something that you just enjoy doing.

Nutrient Density

Nutrient-dense foods are options that provide high amounts of beneficial nutrition per calorie content, meaning they are low in calories but high in nutrients. These nutrients can be in the form of vitamins and minerals, micronutrients, phytochemicals, antioxidants which stimulate healthy cells and destroy bad cells, as well as many other health-promoting components. The most nutrient-dense foods are usually found in the produce area at your local grocery store i.e., fruits and veggies. I'll break down fruits and veggies by category and use simple math to determine how many calories are in one pound of fruits or vegetables. There's a bit more to it when it comes to the type of fruit and the current ripeness, so the below numbers are an approximation per category.

Non-Starchy Vegetables - 100 calories per pound (all leafy greens, peppers, carrots, yellow squash, zucchini, onions, cabbage, mushrooms, celery, asparagus, broccoli, cucumbers, cauliflower, etc...)

Fruit - 300 calories per pound (apples, oranges, melons, mangos, berries, kiwis, lemons, limes, grapes, plums, peaches, etc....)

Starchy Vegetables and Grains- 400-600 calories per pound (potatoes, butternut and acorn squash, corn, oats, whole grains, rice, whole grain pasta, beans, and legumes)

Calorie Density

Foods that contain lots of calories per pound are considered calorically dense, but they usually have little to no nutritional value. There are some calorically dense foods that are considered healthy, like nuts and avocados, while other foods like sugar and fried foods can have negative impacts on your health and weight management goals. That's because these foods don't have the proper nutrients that your body needs. Here's my breakdown of some calorically dense foods per pound.

Avocados -750 calories per pound
Ice cream - 1200 calories per pound
Meat -1200 calories per pound
Bread/Bagel/Wraps - 1400 calories per pound
Cheese and over-the-counter cereals - 1600 calories per pound
Refined sugar, crackers, full buttered popcorn - 1800 calories per pound
Milk chocolate - 2500 calories per pound
Nuts, seeds, and peanut butter - 2800 calories per pound
All oils, and oil popped popcorn - 4000 calories per pound

I used one pound for easy math, but as you can see some foods are very low in calories, but very high in beneficial nutrition, like non-starchy vegetables. While other foods like cheese are very high in calories but offer little to no nutritional value. There are also foods high in calories and high in nutrients like avocados, nuts, and seeds. But the idea is to eat significantly more nutrient dense foods over the calorically dense foods. Once you master this basic concept and once you really change your relationship with food. You shouldn't have any problems losing or maintaining your weight. So, kick calorie counting to the curb and just start enjoying life! In the next chapter we'll discuss the body's internal clock, also known as "The Circadian Rhythm."

Chapter 5

THE CIRCADIAN RHYTHM (INTERNAL CLOCK)

"Three things cannot be long hidden: the
sun, the moon, and the truth." -Buddha

My interpretation for what Buddha meant by
this powerful quote is: We as humans cannot
live independently, as we are all connected to nature
in every single way. Plants need sunlight to release
the foods that are to be provided for human beings
and the other animals who inhabit the earth. Our
eyes become visible to the light during the day, and
they begin to dull when the moon comes out and
darkness settles in. We are hardwired to be more
active and more vibrant during the daylight hours.
This is because our cortisol levels are beginning
to rise and our melatonin levels are starting to
fall. As the moon shines, we naturally gravitate
towards relaxation, because our melatonin levels

are beginning to rise, and our cortisol levels are starting to fall. We are often so relaxed when the sun goes down, we could fall asleep on the couch while watching a Netflix movie and wouldn't notice until someone came to wake us! Finally, the "truth" of the matter is *Mother Nature* is once again perfect in her design. We cannot deny that we have sleep cycles that are in accordance with the risings of the sun and moon.

What Is the Circadian Rhythm?

Did you know that each living creature within nature has its own internal clock or "circadian rhythm?" Circadian rhythms are cycles in the body that occur roughly across a 24-hour period. They are natural processes that take place throughout the day. These rhythms take place everywhere, occurring throughout the natural world in plants and in other animals. They are essential to every organism and occur even in the absence of outside factors. This is a result of certain proteins interacting within the cells of the body, instructing them to be more active or to slow down based on the time of day.

In humans, circadian rhythms cause physical and mental changes within the body, including feelings of wakefulness and sleep. The cycle starts and ends each day depending on the positionings of the sun and moon. To really grasp this concept of your body's circadian rhythm, I'd like to take you back to the birth of a newborn child. When a baby is born and brought home from the hospital, there are times when the parents cannot get a "good night" of rest, because most nights the baby is up crying at 2am. The baby may sometimes sleep most of the day, wake up to eat some food, then it's back to sleep again. This will go on for months or until the baby is around 3-6 months old. The reason a baby sleeps and wakes at odd times is because their circadian rhythm has not been properly programmed or tuned.

A newborn hasn't had enough exposure to the sun and moon, so therefore their internal clock is way off. But as the months and years go by, the child is now sleeping throughout the night like a champ! Newborns need way more sleep than adults because they have the most growing to do. Our bodies grow new cells and repair themselves while we sleep, so it only makes sense that a baby would need the most sleep. As we get older, our body's need for sleep changes significantly. See the below chart for the required amount of sleep a person will need throughout their lifespan to maintain a properly tuned *circadian rhythm.*

Age and sleep needs:

- Newborns (0-2 months) (12-18 hours)
- Infants (3-11 months) (14-15 hours)
- Toddlers (1-3 Years) (12-14 hours)
- Preschoolers (3-5 Years) (11-13 hours)
- School-age children (5-10 years) (10-11 hours)
- Teens (10-17 Years) (8.5-9.5 hours)
- Adults (7-9 hours)

Every cell and organ in our body has their own individual rhythms, so as we experience more of the sun and more of the moon, our cells will begin to reprogram themselves to get in line with the time of day. This is the reason when you're traveling quickly through multiple time zones, you'll experience a condition known as "jet lag." This means your circadian rhythm has been thrown off, so it needs to be reprogrammed by the sun and moon. It will usually take a few days or so for your cells to adjust to the positioning of the sun and moon. But when they adjust, you'll go about your day with normal sleep and wake cycles, which means your rhythm has been restored. However, there are several issues that may alter these naturally occurring circadian rhythms, which could lead to sleep disruptions or other health related issues.

Other examples of circadian rhythms in humans include:

- Hormonal activity
- Body temperature
- Digestion
- Immune function

How Late-Night Snacking Throws off Your Rhythm

As you can see, each cell, system, and organ within your body conforms to or follows a certain set of rules. But for this chapter, I'd like to focus on the process of digestion, other than sleeping patterns. The circadian rhythm has a major impact on digestion and in particular your pancreas. Your pancreas is important for digesting foods and managing blood glucose (sugar) levels, which is used for energy after digestion. Pancreatic hormones help regulate your blood sugar levels, appetite, stimulates stomach acids, and tells your stomach when to empty. After eating a carbohydrate-rich meal, your pancreas will secrete a hormone known as "insulin," which is basically the gatekeeper or security guard for your muscles and liver. Without insulin, the energy we get from the foods we eat wouldn't be able to enter our cells to give us the needed energy to live our lives.

Not only does the circadian rhythm control our sleeping patterns, but it also controls our digestion! When we eat late-night dinners or if we're constantly late-night snacking, it can lead to several gastrointestinal issues. These issues tend to arise because food is not being properly digested and this can lead to excessive acid secretion in your stomach. This is due to your body's metabolism naturally slowing down during the night hours. Our bodies are not as effective at burning calories during the night hours, but it is very effective at burning calories during daylight hours; therefore, eating late at night can lead to weight gain. This is because *Mother Nature* has perfectly designed our circadian rhythm to naturally shut off the pancreas when the sun goes down. And when the moon shines, it's nature's way of telling your body "OK, it's time to start doing some housekeeping and maintenance." Any abnormal cells are removed and discarded by the body's innate ability to naturally heal itself. At night when we sleep, our cells and organs start slowing down and repairing themselves in preparation for the next day, but when we eat late at night, it tricks your pancreas into believing it's daylight hours. This throws off your natural rhythm which can lead to poor sleep, poor digestion, weight gain, and an increased chance of developing a chronic disease or condition.

Homeostasis

Homeostasis is an organism's way of maintaining a stable internal environment suitable for sustaining life. It's your body's way of maintaining balance throughout every cell, system, and organ. We would normally think about homeostasis in terms of the whole body, but individual systems or groups of organs also maintain homeostatic conditions. Therefore, prolonged imbalances in just one of the body's systems can have a huge impact on the homeostatic processes of the entire organism. For example, when it gets cold outside, your body will increase circulation to important organs at the right temperature. It is also responsible for maintaining sugar (glucose) levels within the bloodstream after a meal. As I mentioned earlier, this is the main reason why late-night eating and snacking is very detrimental for optimal health. Maintaining balance is what the body is constantly striving for. But when we give our body's the wrong foods (diesel) at the wrong times (late-night), it can throw off many other systems within our bodies making regaining your health quite the challenge.

Mastering the Art of Intermittent Fasting

Intermittent fasting is an eating pattern where you cycle between periods of eating and not eating. Intermittent fasting is less about what you eat, but more so about the timing of when you eat. Timing is the most important factor when it comes to naturally regaining your health. There are tons of different intermittent fasting methods, all of which split the day, week, or month into eating periods and fasting periods. For the most part, we all *fast* every night when we sleep; therefore, "breakfast" is known as the first meal of the day, because you have broken the "fast."

Intermittent fasting can be as simple as extending that fast a little longer. This can be done by skipping breakfast and eating your first meal at 11am while having your final meal at 7pm. Then you would be officially fasting for 16 hours every day and restricting your eating to an 8-hour window. This is without question the most popular form of intermittent fasting, known as the 16/8 method. In the beginning, it may be challenging to go 16 hours without eating, so others will use the 14/10 method. But if you aren't ready for either of those methods, try giving your body at least 12 hours without food each day by using a 12/12 cycle. Over the span of a couple weeks, your digestive cells and organs will start to reacclimate themselves by shifting their circadian rhythms to match your intermittent fasting window, which in turn steers you closer towards a state of *homeostasis*. Despite what many may think, intermittent fasting is fairly easy to do once you get the hang of it. Many people report feeling better, sleeping better, and having more sustainable energy levels during a fast.

Digestion Times

In the next chapter, I'll get specific on the types of foods you should be eating to maintain great health. These are the things I had to learn about my own *circadian rhythm,* and how my body responded to food based on the time of day. I had to learn what my body needed to function at its best. Before we get into the next chapter, let's finish the topic of digestion. In my weight loss journey, all I ate were plants, so I needed to understand how long it would take for each of the plant food groups to become fully digested, as my goal was to put my body in a state of complete homeostasis. So, if you can understand how long each food group takes to totally digest after consumption, you'll then have a better chance of achieving the goal of optimal health.

For example, digestion of fresh fruits immediately after consumption: One hour in the stomach, one hour in the small intestines, and one hour in the large intestines for a total of three hours.

Digestion of most vegetables immediately after consumption:
Two hours in the stomach, two hours in the small intestines, and two hours in the large intestines for a total of six hours.

Digestion of most grains immediately after consumption: Six hours in the stomach, six hours in the small intestines, six hours in the large intestines for a total of 18 hours.

In closing, your *circadian rhythm* is the master clock within your body that is directly influenced by the light and dark cycles of the sun and moon. Mealtimes also play an important role in the disruption of your *circadian rhythm*. Anything that throws off your natural rhythm, like shiftwork and late-night eating, can and will have major impacts on both your health and wellbeing. As Buddha said, "Three things cannot be long hidden: the sun, the moon, and the *truth!*"

For the next chapter, let's transition into how to heal your body naturally through the power of plant-based nutrition.

Chapter 6

HEALING NATURALLY THROUGH PLANT-BASED NUTRITION

I'm a huge boxing fan, so growing up in the 1980's I watched a ton of Mike Tyson fights. During this time, he was known as the most feared man on the planet. If you've ever watched one of his fights, you'll know exactly what I mean. Most of his fights wouldn't make it out of the first round, because once he hit you, it was lights out! They even made a video game about him; it was called *Mike Tyson's Punch-Out*! So, let me ask you a hypothetical question: if you were to get into the ring with Iron Mike Tyson, and if he were to break your jaw in the very first round, would you go back into the ring with him for round two or would you sit this one out? Would you go back in for round three? My guess is that you wouldn't go back into the ring for the follow-up rounds, because your jaw would clearly need to heal for quite some time. Well, getting back into the ring, round after round with a broken jaw, is essentially what we do as a society every time we consume *diesel fuel* repeatedly, when our body has clearly thrown in the white towel to *stop* the fight!

Your body will throw in the white towel by expressing prolonged inflammation followed by a chronic condition such as high blood pressure, diabetes, heart disease, cancer, ulcerative colitis, rheumatoid arthritis, IBS, strokes, COPD, low energy, obesity, and on and on... But as I mentioned in an earlier chapter, we hardly ever listen to our body. Instead we go back into the ring round after round by repeatedly consuming the wrong fuel sources. Humans typically consume fuel sources like ultra and highly processed junk food, ultra-sweetened beverages, and animal products up to three or more times per day. By doing so, we never actually give our bodies the time it needs to naturally heal itself. This in turn causes your symptoms to worsen until you either become very sick or until your diagnosis becomes terminal.

Construction Site Analogy

Your body wants to heal itself because it is always seeking optimal health, as that is the default state of being, which is known as "homeostasis," or to be within balance. Trust me, it does not want to harbor a disease, extra weight, or a chronic condition. Your body is an extremely complex piece of machinery that has built-in healing mechanisms. For example, have you ever been in your car stuck in traffic due to road construction? I'm willing to bet you have! There are construction workers wearing brightly colored orange or green vests telling you which direction to go, because they're fixing the roads, so therefore no traffic can pass through. They will eventually fix the roads, but to do so they need time and the right equipment. They would never, ever be able to repair the roads with the traffic constantly flowing through, so traffic needs to be redirected or stopped to properly repair the roads. Your body works the exact same way as this construction site analogy: we as human beings are naturally hardwired to heal ourselves.

This means all we have to do is give our body the time and the right environment it needs to thrive, and your body will take care of the rest. But the body's healing power usually never kicks in because we are always digesting food. The speed of how quickly you lose weight or how quickly you heal from a chronic condition, or a disease, is directly proportional to how many healing hours you give your body to repair itself. When we eat the wrong foods, and more importantly when we eat at the wrong times, your body stops the healing process to go digest the food you've just eaten. Digestion takes a huge toll on our system, so natural healing won't kick in unless you've stopped the flow of food. With that, you're probably asking yourself, "well, what is the right environment and how much time do I need to give it?" In the previous chapter, I discussed the importance of your body's own natural circadian rhythm and how long it takes for each specific plant food group to digest. Knowing how long each group takes to digest is very important in helping your body heal. In this chapter, I'll give you the tools you need to properly maximize your eating times and to give your body the best environment to heal itself naturally. So, let's dive in!

Eat Living Foods From Farm to Kitchen

Your body comes directly from nature, so the more natural foods you eat, the better your chances of healing. Make sure the food is living. For example, if you planted a seed in the ground, and if you watered it for a few days, it should grow into a plant. But on the other hand, if you planted something like most processed foods or animal products, the chances of it growing into a plant would be slim to none. My point is this: eat foods that give you life like fruits, vegetables, nuts, seeds, whole grains, and legumes. Your body thrives when it recognizes the food that you're giving it, because it knows exactly what to do with it. Meanwhile, when it comes to things like sodas, candy, cakes, ice cream, sausages, cheeseburgers, donuts, corn dogs, fake vegan burgers, highly refined breads, and most pastas, our body has absolutely no idea what to do with all this low-nutrient *diesel fuel*, so it stores that fuel in our fat cells until it can figure out what to do with it. But as I mentioned earlier, we hardly ever give our body the time it needs to heal, because we are always getting back into the ring to go another round with Mike Tyson.

Eat Whole Foods Directly From Nature

To heal your body naturally, you'll want to eat foods that are wholesome, meaning nature has designed the food perfectly to match our bodies, so don't change it. There's a reason she made avocados instead of avocado oil, potatoes instead of potato chips, dates instead of date sugar, and olives instead of olive oil. All foods that come directly from plants, trees, or the earth are considered wholesome, because they are in their whole, natural forms with their nutrients still intact. *Mother Nature* has already done the planning; she has already designed the foods with the appropriate ratios of protein, fats, and carbohydrates. She also included all the various other plant compounds needed for optimal human health. So, all we must do is listen to what nature is telling us by consuming the natural foods she has perfectly designed.

When we eat the way nature intended, it makes it easier for our bodies to process and eliminate these foods. On the other hand, when we do things like strip away or change the natural nutrient profile of the plant during the refining process just to give it longer shelf life, this can really confuse our systems, because that isn't the way nature intended it. So, eat things like brown rice instead of white rice, as the white rice has been stripped of its bran and germ, which are vital for digestion. Eat whole grains like quinoa, corn, whole oats, and whole wheat pastas instead of refined grains like white bread, white flour, white pasta, crackers, chips, pastries, etc.

Eat Plant-Based

Dairy, fish, eggs, animal flesh, and refined processed foods are not what nature intended for human anatomy. Therefore, consistently filling up on *diesel fuel* while at the pump can lead to lasting negative effects towards overall long-term health. Instead, focus on "eating the rainbow" by eating a colorful variety of fruits and vegetables. Eating the rainbow is a way of eating a balanced diet based on the colors of the food. It is also sometimes called "eat your colors." Foods of a similar color tend to have similar nutrients, as I mentioned earlier, your body is a very complex piece of machinery that needs lots of variety. Each of the colors have different nutrient profiles, so variety is the key. Try aiming to eat 30+ different plants per week to optimize your total health and to boost the body's natural healing properties. There are well over 250,000 edible plants on planet earth, so finding 30 shouldn't be a problem.

My suggestion would be to master the art of making Buddha bowls; these are plant-based meals featuring lots of colorful vegetables served up in a deep bowl. They usually feature a grain as the base, like brown rice or quinoa. You can even make them grain-free by substituting with something like cauliflower rice. After the base, you can add a handful of any leafy greens, beans, chopped non-starchy and/or starchy vegetables, herbs, spices, fruits, avocados, nuts, seeds, sprouts, etc... Your Buddha bowls should look just like the "rainbow," but don't forget to top it off with a beautiful homemade sauce. Your sauce should also consist of plants, including herbs and spices like cilantro, turmeric, and coriander, so this also adds to the total count. These nourishing meals are just little bites of everything thrown into a bowl. You can also make fruit bowls with tons of different fruits like chopped apples, strawberries, blackberries, kiwis, oranges, blueberries, mangos, and bananas, just to name a few! The idea is to eat with tons of variety, and trust me, your body will thank you.

Eat 70% Water-Rich Food and 30% Water-Poor Food

Water-Rich Foods

Many years ago, back when I was in high school, I had to complete a semester of human anatomy. In this class, Mrs. Hester, my teacher, told me the body consisted of approximately 70% water and the other 30% is made of bones, muscle, and mass. In world geography, I learned the earth's surface also consists of approximately 70% water. So, I put two and two together and I once again realized that *Mother Nature* is perfect in her design. So, I thought to myself, "if the earth is 70% water, and my body is also 70% water, shouldn't my food intake consist of 70% water-rich foods?" Now you're probably asking what are water-rich foods? Have you ever heard the term "Eat your water?" These are foods that turn into juice if they're put through a juicing process: foods like pineapples, watermelons, strawberries, cantaloupes, peaches, oranges, cucumbers, spinach, lettuce, zucchini, kale, celery, tomatoes, bell peppers, yellow squash, cabbage, and grapefruits, just to name a few! All of these foods are made of approximately 90% water, so therefore 70% of your plate should consist of these types of foods.

Water-Poor Foods

The remaining 30% of your food intake should consist of foods like grains, oats, nuts, seeds, rice, quinoa, potatoes, breads, pasta, bananas, and beans. Water-poor foods do not produce much water if put through a juicing process. These foods are great, but just like any food, if eaten at the wrong times they can slow down your body's natural healing powers. Earlier, I said your body's ability to heal is solely based on how many healing hours you give it. The healing power only kicks in when you've stopped digesting food. Water-poor foods like grains take much longer to digest than a water rich food like cabbage or leafy greens. If you really want to tap into your body's natural ability to heal, then I would follow the simple philosophy of eating mostly water-rich foods during the morning hours, combine both water-poor and water-rich foods during the afternoon hours, and eat mostly water-rich foods during the evening hours. Consistently timing your meals based on water-poor or water-rich foods can help your body tap into its natural *circadian rhythm,* which in turn steers you closer towards a state of healing and homeostasis.

Chapter 7

DID SOMEONE SAY PROTEIN?

Imagine one day you're out on a nice nature walk when you spot a deer in the woods breastfeeding her newborn, but as you get closer, you notice that she isn't feeding a baby deer, but instead the mother is nursing a baby koala bear! How would you feel about that? Would you ask yourself, "what the hell did I just witness?" or would you think nothing of it and carry on with your walk? I'm guessing you wouldn't be able to shake the image, and it would probably haunt you for weeks on end. But, as the days and weeks go by and as you begin to heal from witnessing such a disturbing image, you decided to go out for another walk, but this time you've decided to choose a different route. On this route, you gaze out into a pasture, and you notice a mother cow breastfeeding a newborn chimpanzee. How would you feel about that? Would you again question *Mother Nature* by asking "what the hell did I just witness?" I surely would!

My point is this: *Mother Nature* does not make mistakes, so if you saw disturbing images like the scenarios I just described, that would probably cause you to question a lot of things. This would most likely be the craziest thing you've ever seen in your life! But there are reasons you'd never see something like the above scenarios in real nature. To get a better understanding as to why you would never see something like these bizarre scenarios, let's first discuss the purpose of milk and why all baby mammals need it, but as we age and gain maturity, the need for milk is no longer needed.

The Milk Protein Hierarchy

Milk is a natural food source for all baby mammals, including humans. We produce milk to feed and nourish our young until they are old enough to chew and digest solid foods on their own. Foods like fruits and vegetables are eaten if you're an herbivore, or dead animal flesh if you're a carnivore like tigers, wolves, and lions. Milk's sole purpose is to make a baby mammal grow into a bigger mammal, as milk has all the necessary nutrients the baby will ever need. But here's where nature drew a line in the sand: *Mother Nature* says depending on how fast that mammal grows, this and this alone will determine how much protein is encased within its milk. For example, it only takes a rat or mouse about three weeks from its birth to reach a good size to where it can fend for itself, but it only takes six months for that rat to reach full adulthood. On the other hand, it takes human beings about 18 years to reach full adulthood. A glass of rat milk has 10 times more protein per gram than that of human milk. So, the question is, "what role does protein play in the growth process?"

All mammals need protein to survive, as it is responsible for good immune health, energy, regulating the body's processes, as well as helping to balance fluids. But the main thing protein does is that it builds and repairs new cells to make strong muscles and bones. It's also responsible for making a baby grow. Protein is broken down into 20 individual building blocks known as Branched-Chain Amino Acids. Of these 20, there are 8-9 essential amino acids that cannot be made by the human body, and therefore, we need to get those amino acids from the foods we eat. But this still doesn't answer the question as to why a tiny mouse or rat would have 10 times more protein in its milk than that of human milk. Well, the answer is simple: *Mother Nature* designed it that way, she knows that rats reach their full adulthood by the time they're six months old, so she specifically encased large amounts of protein and fat within the rat's milk to compensate for how fast the animal grows.

On the other hand, she specifically designed human milk to have significantly less protein and fat, because she knows that humans grow at a MUCH slower rate than rats. So, with that in mind, she purposefully designed human milk to have lower amounts of protein. As a matter-of-fact, human breast milk has about the lowest percentage of protein per gram than that of any other species on the planet, because of our slow rate of growth. For example, when we graduate from high school our parents can't wait to send us off to college or to the military, because they couldn't wait to finally become "empty nesters!" They'll sit you down and say something like this: "Well, you're 18 years old and you are officially an adult, so get out there and go enjoy your life!" So, with this in mind, Mother Nature didn't put large amounts of protein within our nutrition, because 18 years is quite a long time.

Here's another example: 100 grams of whole cow's milk has about 3.3 grams of protein while human milk only has 1.3 grams of protein per 100 grams. Growing calves need more protein to enable them to grow quickly, as it takes about two years for a calf to become a full-sized cow. While human infants, on the other hand, need less protein and more fat because most of the energy we expend is primarily related to the development of our brains, spinal cord, and nerves. Humans have huge brains, so the proper amounts of healthy fats like the ones we get from fruits and veggies are ideal for proper brain development and health.

The proteins found in cow's milk have a completely different ratio of macro and micronutrients compared to that of human milk. For example, cow's milk has two proteins called casein and whey, and both these proteins contribute to the thickness and creaminess of the milk along with tons of saturated fat. The higher saturated fat content in cow's milk allows us to make thick and great tasting ice cream, while human milk, on the other hand, would be *terrible* for making ice cream, because human milk has a completely different ratio of fats, protein, and carbohydrates. Cow's milk has a casein protein ratio of 80%, while human milk comes in around 40% casein. A cow doubles in size every 40 days while human babies double in size every 180 days. Therefore, *Mother Nature* designed cow's milk to have much more protein than that of human milk. The protein *casein* is also very difficult for humans to digest, so therefore human milk has less protein, but has more carbohydrates and fats.

As I mentioned earlier, *Mother Nature* does not make mistakes, so the protein content found in human milk is more sustainable for human babies. Lower protein intake is less taxing on the kidneys of a developing infant. As humans become adults, we still need protein for strong muscles and bone repair, but if you're not trying to become a bodybuilder or super-athlete, there is no need to go crazy about how much protein you're consuming.

Just stick to eating your natural diet filled with a variety of whole plant foods and you'll do just fine. As you'll discover in the next chapter, "Marketing is One Hell of a Thing," the most protein you'll ever need is when you're in the growing phase of adolescence and youth, because that's when you're in the bulk of your growing. Once you become an adult, your brain sends a signal to the rest of your body, saying the growth process is complete, it's time to stop growing, and it is now time to maintain a great balance between healthy carbohydrates, fats, and protein. As I mentioned earlier, the body loves being in a state of *homeostasis*.

Plant vs. Animal Protein

Plant Protein

For the most part, animal proteins like meat, dairy, and eggs contain all 20 of the essential amino acids from protein. Meat is known as a complete protein source, while plant-based proteins like beans, nuts, seeds, whole grains, and soy are rich in some amino acids, but may lack some of the other essential acids. The human body does not store excess protein, so living a plant-based lifestyle calls for lots of *variety*. You will not get all the required amino acids if you're just keeping it *extremely* simple; the idea is variety, variety, variety. In the last chapter, I spoke about "eating the rainbow" by aiming to eat 30+ different plants per week. This is nature's way of saying "I put over 250,000+ edible plants on this planet for a reason," and that reason is called "variety." When you combine and eat lots of different plants, you are now getting all the essential amino acids (protein) that is required. So, again, if you're eating with variety and getting in enough calories, then I wouldn't worry too much about how much protein you're consuming. Plant protein sources are also rich in disease fighting antioxidants, low in saturated fats, high in fiber, and optimally designed for human physiology.

Animal Protein

Animal proteins are eggs, dairy, and meats such as beef, pork, poultry, racoons, seafood, deer, goat, and alligator (and yes, I did say racoons!). Meat is known as a complete, high-quality protein source containing all the essential amino acids your body needs for optimal health. Your body can make some amino acids by itself, but you must get the remaining nine from your diet, AKA "essential amino acids." But, when I started my vegan journey, I questioned that theory and I started asking myself, "how essential are these animal proteins, and do I really need them to survive?" You see, I really loved eating eggs; during the holidays my sister and niece would make the most amazing deviled eggs, and I would make a big pot of scrambled eggs for my entire family. But what I really loved most was making the biggest and cheesiest egg omelet that you could ever imagine. But in my research, I discovered what an egg is and where it comes from, so I decided the six grams of protein along with all the artery clogging and saturated fat from just one egg was not worth my efforts nor my health.

Allow me to elaborate on what an egg is and where they come from. Eggs are the unfertilized reproductive system of hen (female chicken). During ovulation, a yellow, mature egg yolk is secreted from the ovary of the hen. It then travels through the oviduct (similar to the human fallopian tubes) where it is accompanied by a substance called albumen (egg white), which guards and protects the yolk all the way through the oviduct. The yolk travels until it reaches the shell gland (or uterus), where the shell is formed mostly from a compound called "calcium carbonate"; this is because the hen mobilizes or takes about 10% of the *calcium* from its own bones to make the eggshell. The final stage of the process is the birth canal or vagina, which is about 4-5 inches long. The vagina does not play a big part in the formation of the egg, but it's very important for laying the eggs, because it has the muscles to help push the egg out of the hen's body. If the egg was fertilized during the process by a rooster (male chicken), the egg will hatch into a yellow baby chicken or chick. If the egg was not fertilized, it is taken and used for human consumption.

So, in essence, an egg is the unfertilized reproductive system of a female chicken. When we crack open to fry an egg, the yellow yolk is what would have been a yellow baby chick, and the egg whites are the protective compound known as "albumen," which protects the yolk so that it makes it all the way to the end of the birth canal or vagina. Once I learned the true natural origins of this specific animal protein, I decided to cut ties with eggs all together. I thought to myself, "there wasn't a chance in hell that I was going to have another egg, because I know exactly what it is and where it came from." I also asked myself, "Was *Mother Nature* flawed in her design?" Because I thought, "why the hell would she have me eating the reproductive system of a chicken to reach my daily protein needs?" I almost had to call Child Protective Services (CPS) once again, because I thought, "what type of mother would do something so heinous!"

Are You Really Lactose Intolerant?

On average, 65-70% of the world's adult population is lactose intolerant. The prevalence of lactose intolerance varies amongst different ethnicities. It is most common in African Americans, Hispanics/Latinos, and Asians. It is least prevalent in people of

European descent. So, the question is why is more than half of the world's adult population allergic to lactose? Well, let's dive into it. L*actose* is a sugar within milk, and when we are babies we need lactose. Babies can easily break down lactose into its individual components so that it can be used by the baby for energy and growth. Babies produce lots of a specialized enzyme called "lactase," which is responsible for breaking down the lactose to easily digest the milk. Our problems with lactose start when we get older and become adults, because the older we get, the fewer "lactase" enzymes our body produces, which makes breaking down *lactose* very difficult. So it isn't that you're lactose intolerant, it's more so that you are not a baby, and in particular, you are not a baby cow. I know how difficult it is to give up cheese because as I mentioned earlier, I had no intentions of ever giving up my double cheeseburgers with extra pickles. Now I know cheese is the absolute worst thing on the planet for an adult to consume because of what it does to your body. It is also one of the most addictive substances on the planet. But now I totally understand what cheese is and where it comes from.

In an earlier chapter, I mentioned an animal product called "rennet" which is an enzyme primarily used in the production of cheese. Allow me to explain what this enzyme is and how it's used. This enzyme is extracted from the inner parts of the fourth stomach of an unweaned baby cow. Baby cows produce this enzyme to break down their mother's milk, similar to "lactase" in humans. After the baby calf is slaughtered then turned into veal, that enzyme is removed from its stomach to make cheese. It is used in the production of cheese as a "curdling" agent to break down the milk's *protein* which allows the cheese to harden. It's also what makes the cheese gooey! Without this specialized enzyme, the milk wouldn't turn from a liquid to a solid. So, once I figured out that most cheese is made from a specialized enzyme produced from the stomach of an unweaned baby cow, I decided to ditch the cheese altogether. I gave up my double cheeseburgers with extra pickles because I discovered what can happen when you consume too much of the wrong protein sources.

Remember dairy/milk is responsible for making things grow, so too much as an adult can cause the wrong things to grow within your cells. Your cells are receiving the signal from milk to grow, but as an adult you don't want things to grow because you've already reached full adulthood. So, what grows instead? Things like fat and cancer cells begin to grow. Animal protein causes your body to produce more of a hormone called IGF-1 or "insulin like growth factor 1," which is an anabolic hormone that has the role of stimulating growth, and to a lesser degree, it supports the maintenance of normal blood sugar (insulin) levels and a healthy metabolism. There have been many studies identifying a very powerful link between milk and various forms of cancer. So, if you can, it may be best to avoid milk and cheese altogether, or at a minimum, drastically cut down on your intake. Studies are inconclusive; however, more research is being conducted to better understand the link. As I mentioned in the opening story of this chapter, "It would probably be the craziest thing you've ever witnessed in life if you ran across a baby koala bear being breastfed by a mother deer."

Well, the moral of that story was: this is what we as human beings do every time we grab that glass of cow's milk or bite into a succulent piece of cheese. But if it's *protein* we're after, then a much better option would be to drink a nice tall glass rat's milk over cow's milk, because that stuff is loaded- and I mean LOADED- with way more *protein* than that of any other species on this planet. So, again it isn't that you're lactose intolerant, it's simply because you are not a baby, and in particular, you are not a baby cow!

Chapter 8

MARKETING IS ONE HELL OF A THING

In today's fast-paced modern world, you don't have to look very far to find the latest advertising and marketing campaigns naming the newest foods coming to market. Whether you're turning on your television, listening to the radio or a podcast, driving down the highway in your car, or twisting the throttle on your sport bike, you can be pretty much guaranteed to see or hear some form of advertisements. Food companies spend billions of dollars every year to market anything and everything that you could ever imagine. Their sole purpose is getting "you," the consumer, to take bait by purchasing their products. As I've mentioned several times in this book, I used to love- and I mean LOVE- going to the McDonald's™ drive-thru several times per week to grab my favorite: a double cheeseburger with extra pickles and a small fry.

On average, I would pay $2.50 for the combo, and if I wanted to add the additional drink, the total would be around $3.50. I knew that was all I needed to satisfy my cravings, then I would be off to my daily routine. I never questioned the price, I just thought to myself, "hey, that price seems fair to me!" There would often be days when I'd double up by traveling over to Burger King™ to also grab a double cheeseburger with extra pickles and a small fry with a drink for a similar price. If you were to know anything about me, it is that I had an infatuation with these cheeseburgers. You would know that these burgers were a staple in my daily diet and nutrition. So the fact that I could get an entire meal with my favorite foods at McDonald's and Burger King for less than $4 was a joy to my soul. I used to say, "you can't beat these prices; I *love* the dollar menu!" Every time I would see a commercial or hear about the dollar menu on the radio, my pleasure receptors would kick into high gear and I'd be at the nearest drive-thru, because I just couldn't resist the urge to have a cheeseburger.

But once I gave up the burgers and made the transition over to a plant-based vegan lifestyle, I started to spend a lot more time at the supermarket and in the produce aisle. Now I'm shopping for things like brightly colored fruits and vegetables. One fruit in particular is very bright in color and is extremely nutritious, that fruit is called a Dragon fruit. No, I'm not referring to the type of dragons that you may see on *Game of Thrones;* I'm referring to a fruit low in calories and packed with essential vitamins and minerals. It also contains a substantial amount of dietary fiber, iron, and magnesium, along with lots of cancer-fighting phytonutrients, like antioxidants. I'm now on a natural journey, and learning about all the health benefits of plant-based nutrition also made my soul very happy.

But what didn't make my soul happy was finding out that one dragon fruit that can easily fit into the palm of my hand could cost on average around $6-7. Yet, I could go over to McDonalds or Burger King and purchase an entire meal filled with nutritionally devoid animal products for less than $4. I said to myself, "that doesn't make any sense." I thought, "how could I get an entire meal at a low cost when I pull up to the drive-thru at a fast-food joint, but a single brightly colored dragon fruit costs around 7 bucks?" So, I did some digging, and I discovered the US government gives subsidies to both the meat and dairy industries to keep the prices low and affordable when the products come to market. They also subsidize the fruit and vegetable industries, but there's a huge difference in how much money each industry gets.

For example, there are 38,000,000,000 (that's 38 billion) dollars per year in government subsidies that go to the meat, dairy, and egg industries while the fruit and vegetable industry only receives 20,000,000. That's 20 million versus 38 billion. That's a HUGE disparity, so this is the reason I used to practically live at the fast food drive-thru with limited to no impact on my pockets. Now I understand why fruits and vegetables tend to cost SO much more when I go to the produce aisle at the local Farmer's Market. Not only is there a huge disparity in the amount of money spent by the government to push these unhealthy products, but there are billions of dollars spent each year by the food industry to chemically activate the dopamine (pleasure) receptors in your brain to keep you coming back for more.

So, as you can imagine, this was quite literally a "mind-boggling" discovery. These highly refined, diesel-fueled products activate our dopamine receptors, similar to powerful drugs like opioids, alcohol, cocaine, and heroin. They are designed this way to keep you coming back for more, or until you've become completely hooked. This is the reason I couldn't resist going to the drive-thru for a double cheeseburger; I just had to have one! The food industry knows exactly how to produce and market the perfect combination of sugar, salt, and fat that will send your taste buds and pleasure receptors into overdrive.

Fast Food Restaurants

A few years ago, around the time I was in the worst shape of my life, I saw a commercial advertising the newest chicken sandwich at KFC™. So, my wife and I jumped in the car to go check it out. We were destined to have this sandwich, because the advertisement was SO spot on that we couldn't hardly resist! Allow me to describe word for word what an article written by www.eatthis.com from February of 2020 wrote. Once you read the description, you'll understand why we had to immediately have this sandwich. And I quote: "Mealtime is about to be even more finger-lickin' good with the new KFC donut sandwich. Start your day—or literally any meal—off on the right foot with KFC's sweet-meets-savory dish: the Kentucky Fried Chicken & Donuts. You could get this epic combination served separately in a basket, but why go that route when you can also have it as a sandwich? Yes, we said a sandwich! Imagine having fried chicken nestled between two hot, glazed donuts for a bite that's a little bit breakfast, a little bit of lunch, and a whole lot of flavor. You won't have to daydream much longer, as you can experience this **blissfulness** at your local KFC as early as next week."

So, I said to myself "that has to be absolutely the worst idea I've ever seen or heard of for a chicken sandwich!" But the pleasure receptors in my brain kicked into high gear, and I just couldn't stop thinking about donuts and chicken joining forces together on a sandwich. But here's the thing: even though I initially thought the sandwich was a terrible idea, I just couldn't resist the urge to go buy one, because I knew that perfectly manufactured combination of sugar, salt, and fat would temporarily satisfy my cravings and that it would drive me to want more! When I arrived, the cashier asked if I wanted fries with my sandwich, and I said, "hell yes, give me those fries too!" Well, during the eating of this sandwich, my initial intuition was correct. I suffered through every bite of this sandwich, because the richness was just too much for me to handle. I said to myself, "yup, this has to be the worst chicken sandwich I've ever eaten in my life!" The moral of that story was even though I initially thought it was a terrible idea for a chicken sandwich, I still needed to try it because the marketing was just so beautifully done. Hence the name of this chapter "Marketing is One Hell of a Thing."

Children Are Like Sponges

With childhood obesity on the rise in the US, and according to a study conducted between the years 2017-2020 by the CDC, it says that approximately 22% of children in the US between the ages of 12-19 years old are either overweight or obese. Childhood

Type 2 diabetes, hypertension, and heart disease are all on a steep incline. So, the question needs to be, "why is childhood obesity on the rise and why are so many kids suffering from diabetes and hypertension?" There have been more studies that say by the time the kids of this generation reach the age of 10, their arteries are already clogged and filled with cholesterol and plaque. This is because they are eating all the products being advertised and marketed on the radio and television. As I mentioned in Chapter 2, these products are not *real food;* they have the look, feel, and taste of *real food*. But the truth of the matter is these products are nothing more than high-octane diesel fuel, devoid of any real nutritional value. With marketing and the world being so fast-paced, it's easy to understand how children can also get caught in the vicious cycle of *yo-yo dieting*.

Our children never really get to experience what real, whole, natural food is. They are rarely taught what true health is, and fruits and vegetables are almost never mentioned. Instead, they are subliminally subjected to everything they see on TV, or they'll watch what their parents eat and mimic that same behavior. When this behavior is mimicked, children will experience the same common diseases as most adults. When children eat mostly processed food, dairy, and animal products, it can and will trigger the *"werewolf curse."* However, as I mentioned earlier, the werewolf gene can stay dormant by never rearing its ugly head if we simply teach our children to stay away from these gene-triggering products.

Marketing of the Latest FDA Approved Drugs

When it comes to pharmaceuticals, the US is by far at the top of the list when it compares to the rest of the world for the sale, purchase, and revenue generated by some of these powerful drugs. But, I don't mean powerful in a good way. For example, did you know that the U.S. Pharmaceutical Industry earned $550 billion in annual revenue in 2021? According to a study conducted by www.zippia.com, which was published in September 2022, those earnings are nearly double what they were a decade ago. Also in 2021, there were about 4.7 billion prescriptions dispensed in the United States. But the stat that really blows my mind is knowing that over 1 million children under the age of five are being prescribed one or more psychotropic drugs. They are being prescribed stimulants, antidepressants, antipsychotics, mood stabilizers, and anxiolytics to treat their anxiety disorders. So, the question must be raised. "Are these drugs really needed for our children or is there an alternative?" Imagine what would happen if instead of using pills and medications to treat our diseases and disorders.

What would happen if we prescribed plants as our medicine?

When I received my heart disease and pre-diabetes diagnosis, I refused to take the prescribed cholesterol statins. As I mentioned in an earlier chapter, I was taught a very valuable lesson on a cruise by one of the excursion tour guides. He said, "we don't get our medicine from a pharmacy; we get our medicine from the land." With that philosophy in mind, I reversed both those conditions without taking any medications. So, what would happen if a Whole-Foods, Plant-Based Natural Diet and Lifestyle were advertised and prescribed instead of over-the-counter drugs and prescription medications? In my opinion, if that were to happen, the entire medical system would crumble. Hospitals would go bankrupt, bypass and stent procedures would be a thing of the past, Type 2 Diabetes would cease to exist, and there would be less cancer.

These pharmaceutical companies are making lots of money, but at what expense? It's at the expense of the people! If you go into your doctor's office and if you're prescribed a medicine, they will most likely tell you that you'll have to take that medication for the rest of your life. So then ask yourself, "is taking medication or a drug for a condition that can either be improved upon or totally reversed really something that you want to do for the rest of your life?" Or is simply changing what's at the end of your fork a better option?

ADOPTING THE RIGHT MINDSET

Listen, during the writing of this book I wanted to create an experience for you by taking you on a journey and into the mind of a self-proclaimed "*mad scientist.*" I wanted you to experience all the highs and lows that lead me to being the person that I am today. Plants changed my body, but I first needed to adopt the right mindset. So, in this final chapter I wanted to fill it with advice I would have given to my younger self if I could relive my 30s, because my health problems began literally the day I turned 40!

Adopting the Right Mindset

I would say, "You can change your lifestyle at any age, it doesn't matter if you're a toddler or 100 years old." I would often hear stories of people saying once you get older, it's much harder to maintain your health, and that it's only inevitable to end up fat, out of shape, and sick. And that you're destined to have a *"dad bod"* once you get older. Now I know that health is not determined by age and that you should feel good in your own skin, no matter how old you are! And that it's never too late to start something new. I would say, "you're always in control of your health and age does not define the choices you make." Embrace new challenges and learn from your mistakes and never give up on anything that you're passionate about. Get inspired from the success of others; if they can do it, then so can you. During my years of *yo-yo dieting,* I would lose the weight only to gain it back. I would often tell myself, "I can't do this anymore, this sucks." I wanted to lose the weight so badly, but I just didn't know how to, so I always would go back to what I knew and what was comfortable for me.

Now I would say, "Your weight loss success or failure doesn't matter, all I want is to know that you've given it your best. If you do something, do it at 100%." I would tell myself to never weigh your food, count calories or macros. Not only does that not help you in living a healthy and balanced lifestyle, but instead it just contributes to more stress, guilt, confusion, and just being overwhelmed by food. I would say only eat the food that *Mother Nature* herself has provided for you. Eat mostly plants, and fill up on unleaded fuel, not the diesel fuel. Start creating habits around your daily activities. I would tell myself to slowly transition into a plant-based lifestyle to lose the weight naturally and keep it off, because as I mentioned earlier, your body literally wants to heal. So, when you get older, you don't have to fall under those same cliches of it only being inevitable to be fat, out of shape, and sick. I would say when you turn 40 years old you should look and feel like you're 20.

When I started my plant-based journey, I had no intentions of being back to my high school weight. I only wanted to be free of heart disease and pre-diabetes. But in doing so, I realized that it's true; your body just wants to heal. All I did was change my fuel source from diesel to unleaded, and I gave my body the time it needed to heal itself naturally. I didn't change my workouts, but I was more consistent in my schedule. I made it my purpose to get up to move daily. I pushed myself to stay consistent and focused. I would have saved myself lots of years of "yo-yo dieting" had I just kept it super simple by just eating *real food*.

Become Your Own Doctor

I often see billboards that say, "when the doctor looks like this, forget the apples." The board has a picture of a nice-looking doctor smiling with a stethoscope. The advertisement is implying that a doctor can heal you from your ailments, so therefore the eating of plants is not important. As I mentioned earlier, "Marketing is one hell of a thing." The notion of doctors healing you couldn't be further from the truth. I'm not telling you *not* to listen to your doctor, but my advice would be to do your own research and become your own doctor.

Doctors are great when we really need them, but just like the analogy I gave you about the 4x100 relay, let's only use them for a short period of time or only when necessary.

My goal is to make going to the doctor's office to treat common diseases like some of the ones I've mentioned in this book obsolete, or only to be used in cases of emergency. Doctors can treat your symptoms, but they can't take care of you. That responsibility must fall solely upon you. I was prescribed a statin by my doctor for my soaring cholesterol numbers, but I was so determined to find out the truth behind what it was that I would be putting into my body. So, I decided to turn down his offer and instead I became my own doctor.

In my studies, I've learned there are only two types of doctors: those who have picked up the literature about how plants can heal the body, and those who have not! Have you ever heard the saying, "I want to add years to my life?" I thought, "How would adding years to my life be beneficial for me if I'm taking medications for heart disease every single day?" I thought to myself "that's not freedom, why would I want to add years to my life, yet I'm needing to take this medication to treat my illness."

Instead, when I'm old and gray, I want to *add life to my years* free of medications. I still want to have the ability to be active and still able to run like a kid.

The benefits of exercising with regularity or just simply being active on a regular basis is very important for your long-term overall health. Exercise has always been the miracle cure we've always had, but for far too long we've neglected to take advantage of it, and we've failed to reach our recommended dose. As a result, your health is now suffering because of a sedentary lifestyle and poor food choices. Let the truth be told, that it doesn't matter your age, there is strong scientific evidence that being physically active can help you lead a healthier and happier life. Studies have shown that people who exercise regularly have a lower risk of developing many of the common long-term (chronic) conditions, like heart disease, Type 2 Diabetes, strokes, and some cancers.

How Determined Are You?

What is your "why?" What drives you to get out of the bed each morning? If you could visualize your determination, how would it look? Through my years of *yo-yo dieting,* I understand how hard it is to lose weight and how difficult it is to consistently stay motivated. But here's the thing about that: you don't have to be motivated 100% of the time, but you can be disciplined 100% of the time. Weight loss and regaining your health is not impossible. Weight loss is hard, but hard is not the same as impossible. Being overweight is equally as hard, so you have to make the decision and choose your hard. But the biggest secret to losing weight is believing you can do it, and realizing that it's not going to happen overnight.

Instead, focus on eating the foods that most serve your mental and physical well-being. Now I realize the causes and effects of making food choices and how those choices affect your health. In my journey to regain my health, I learned that it's your level of discipline that will determine your level of success. Society doesn't make living a plant-based lifestyle easy. For example, when I travel, I'll often use an app on my phone to locate a nice plant-based vegan restaurant, or at least a place that has vegan options, because plants are not what's on the advertisement billboards. So it can sometimes turn into quite the adventure. Often, I'll stop by the local grocery store to grab a bunch of fresh fruits and veggies to stock my hotel fridge. But going through these extra lengths does not bother me, because I decided to choose my health over convenience. My purpose is fueled by my passion.

I think about my "why," so when it gets hard to keep going, let that "why" be your strength. As some time passes and whether you have success or whether you fail, you can still look back to see how far you've come from where you started. To fail simply means it is your *"first attempt in learning."* Sometimes, whatever you're doing to reach your goals may not be working, so you must set a very specific vision, but be OPEN to it unfolding in different ways. Sometimes, we forget that baby steps still move us forward, taking the proper actions towards your goals is the only thing holding you back from reaching your full potential.

Don't wait for tomorrow to start building the healthy lifestyle habits that you've always dreamt of; start now! Saying "because I want this" can often be enough motivation. Being motivated will get you started, but discipline keeps you moving. Master your daily routine so that you can master your success. When it came to finally losing the weight and regaining my health, I had to stop lying to myself about not having enough time. I had all the time that was required, all I had to do was make the time to master my routine and the success followed. When your distractions no longer distract you, that's called *discipline*. The harder you work for something, the greater you'll feel when you achieve it.

Let Nature Be Your Guide

I started this book with The Laws of Nature by explaining the three special diets for each of the living species that inhabit the earth. I ended the book with "Marketing is One Hell of a Thing." So, when the going gets tough, and when the tough gets going, and when you start getting confused by all the different marketing campaigns, just remember there is *one thing* that will reign supreme over any subliminal messages made by marketing campaigns or by any conflicting advice given to you by a man, and that is to "listen to what *Mother Nature* says, because she is, and always will be, ***perfect*** in her design."

ABOUT THE AUTHOR

Kelley started his career in the US Navy. His last three years in the military were spent as an instructor at the US Naval Academy in Annapolis, MD, where he became a certified instructor and Master Training Specialist. After transitioning out of the military, he became a Product Specialist within the oil and gas industry, conducting training classes for companies like Shell, ExxonMobil, BP, and Chevron. He trained their personnel on how to commission, operate, troubleshoot, and fix their machinery. During that time, he gained a ton of weight, and his health began to spiral out of control. He eventually became obese and was later diagnosed with both prediabetes and heart disease at the very same doctor's visit. He was so determined to reverse the misfortunes of his own health that he went back to school and became a Certified Holistic Nutritionist with a specialty in plant-based medicine. He lost nearly 70 pounds in less than a year and reversed all his health conditions by using the power of plant-based nutrition. In February of 2022, he started his company, One Determined Vegan, where he now helps and teaches his clients how to harness the power of nature to naturally heal their bodies from chronic disease using plant-based nutrition.

Learn more at: OneDeterminedVegan.com

Made in United States
North Haven, CT
25 February 2024

49191257R10079